# GYNECOLOGIC
# PEARLS

# GYNECOLOGIC PEARLS

*Second Edition*

## MICHAEL D. BENSON, MD, FACOG

Lecturer
Department of Obstetrics and Gynecology
Northwestern University Medical School
Chicago, Illinois

**F. A. DAVIS COMPANY** • Philadelphia

F. A. Davis Company
1915 Arch Street
Philadelphia, PA 19103

Printed in Canada

List digit indicates print number: 10 9 8 7 6 5 4 3 2 1

*Acquisitions Editor:* Robert W. Reinhardt
*Developmental Editor:* Bernice M. Wissler
*Cover Designer:* Louis J. Forgione

As new scientific information becomes available through basic and clinical
research, recommended treatments and drug therapies undergo changes.
The author(s) and publisher have done everything possible to make this book
accurate, up to date, and in accord with accepted standards at the time of
publication. The authors, editors, and publisher are not responsible for errors or omissions or for consequences from application of the book, and
make no warranty, expressed or implied, in regard to the contents of the
book. Any practice described in this book should be applied by the reader in
accordance with professional standards of care used in regard to the unique
circumstances that may apply in each situation. The reader is advised always
to check product information (package inserts) for changes and new information regarding dose and contraindications before administering any drug.
Caution is especially urged when using new or infrequently ordered drugs.

**Library of Congress Cataloging-in-Publication Data**

Benson, Michael D.
    Gynecologic pearls / Michael D. Benson. — 2nd ed.
        p. cm.
    Includes bibliographical references and index.
    ISBN 0-8036-0502-1 (pbk.)
    1. Gynecology—Handbooks, manuals, etc. 2. Generative organs,
Female—Diseases—Handbooks, manuals, etc. I. Title.
    [DNLM: 1. Genital Diseases, Female—handbooks. 2. Contraception—
handbooks. WP 39 B4739g 2000]
    RG110.B47 2000
    618.1—dc21                                              99-055261

# Preface

My editors at F. A. Davis and I are particularly pleased with this new edition of *Gynecologic Pearls*. It has been completely reorganized and rewritten to cover a broader amount of material in the same space. In keeping with the pattern established by its companion book, *Obstetrical Pearls,* the material has been divided into geographic regions of the hospital such as the general gynecology clinic, surgery, and subspecialty clinics. In this way, all the relevant information for a particular activity in the clinical rotation is quickly available in one section. This edition has some completely new material such as discussions on Bartholin duct abscesses, toxic shock syndrome, the treatment of prolapse and urinary incontinence, and examples of surgical dictation.

In the 4 years since the first edition was published, the specialty of gynecology has changed incredibly. New procedures such as balloon endometrial ablation and hysterosonograms are now routine in gynecologic practice. Although oral contraceptives have been around for nearly 40 years, several new formulations have emerged and there is a new indication—the treatment of acne. Where one progestational agent was available 4 years ago, three can be used at the time of this edition. Perhaps one of the most spectacular advances in medicine of all time is also one of the least recognized: the enormous strides in the treatment of HIV. With combination therapy, the mortality rates in Western countries are dropping so quickly that the literature cannot keep up. It is truly an exciting time to be a physician.

In preparing this book, as for all volumes in this series, the publisher and I have tried to:

- Cover 95% of what is encountered during a medical school rotation and the first two years of a gynecology residency
- Focus on meaningful information so that 95% of what appears in the book will be encountered during a clinical rotation
- Make the book brief enough to be read cover to cover in 3 or 4 hours.

It is simply not possible to perform well or absorb much out of a clinical rotation if one has to read a thousand-page text just to have some idea of what is going on. For this reason, we believe that the Pearls series fills a vital role in medical education.

**Michael D. Benson, MD, FACOG**
Deerfield, Illinois

# Contents

**PART 1—THE GYNECOLOGY CLINIC**  1

CHAPTER 1
THE GYNECOLOGIC HISTORY
AND PHYSICAL .............................................  3
Gynecologic Anatomy   3
Gynecologic History   6
Pelvic Examination   7
Making the Exam More Bearable   9
Female Circumcision   10

CHAPTER 2
MENSTRUATION AND ABNORMAL
BLEEDING .......................................................  12
The Menstrual Cycle   12
Menarche and Puberty   15
Feminine Hygiene   18
Dysmenorrhea   20
Infrequent Menstruation   21
Polycystic Ovarian Syndrome (PCOS)   23
Excessive Bleeding   24
First-Trimester Bleeding   27

CHAPTER 3
CONTRACEPTION .........................................  30
The Combination Oral Contraceptive Pill   30
The "Morning-After" Pill   41
Progestin-Only Contraceptives   41

The Intrauterine Device   44
Spermicides and Barrier Methods   49
Periodic Abstinence   55
Female Sterilization   55
Male Sterilization   58
Abortion   59
Contraceptive Safety and Effectiveness   65

CHAPTER 4
VULVAR AND VAGINAL COMPLAINTS ......   68
Vulvar Irritation   68
Vaginal Discharge   72
Pain on Intercourse (Dyspareunia)   74
Bartholin Duct Abscess   74
Retained Tampon   76
Toxic Shock Syndrome   76

CHAPTER 5
MISCELLANEOUS GYNECOLOGIC
PROBLEMS ......................................................   77
Premenstrual Syndrome   77
Decreased Libido   79
Galactorrhea   79
Hirsutism   82
Pelvic Pain   84

PART 2—SPECIALTY CLINICS          85

CHAPTER 6
UROGYNECOLOGY CLINIC   87
Prolapse   87
Urinary Incontinence   89

CHAPTER 7
SEXUALLY TRANSMITTED DISEASE
CLINIC ...........................................................   100
An Inventory of Sexually Transmitted
Diseases   100
Hepatitis B   108
Genital Herpes Infection   111
Human Immunodeficiency Virus Infection   113
Pelvic Inflammatory Disease   117
Syphilis   120

**CHAPTER 8**
COLPOSCOPY CLINIC .................................... 125
  Microscopic Anatomy of the Cervix   125
  Human Papillomavirus   126
  Biology of Cervical Intraepithelial Neoplasia   129
  Cervical Cytology   130
  Follow-up of Abnormal Pap Smears   132
  Treatment of Squamous Intraepithelial
    Lesions   136

**CHAPTER 9**
THE MENOPAUSE CLINIC ........................... 141
  Hormone Replacement Therapy   142
  Osteoporosis   147
  Assessment of Postmenopausal Bleeding   149
  Premature Ovarian Failure   150

**CHAPTER 10**
REPRODUCTIVE ENDOCRINOLOGY
CLINIC ........................................................... 151
  Evaluation of the Infertile Couple   152
  Treatment of Infertility   156
  Endometriosis   161

**CHAPTER 11**
THE GYNECOLOGIC ONCOLOGY
CLINIC ........................................................... 165
  Vulvar Neoplasms   165
  Cervical Cancer   167
  Uterine Neoplasms   167
  Ovarian Neoplasms   171
  Gestational Trophoblastic Disease   173
  Breast Disease   174

**PART 3—THE OPERATING ROOM**    **181**

**CHAPTER 12**
SURGICAL INSTRUMENTS, MATERIALS,
AND TECHNIQUES ...................................... 183
  Commonly Used Surgical Instruments, Sutures,
    and Needles   183
  Laparoscopic Instruments   185
  Lasers and Electrosurgical Devices   187
  Surgical Technique   189

**CHAPTER 13**
SPECIFIC OPERATIONS ............................. 190
Abdominal Hysterectomy and Bilateral
  Salpingo-Oophorectomy 190
Vaginal Hysterectomy 194
Laparoscopy 196
Dilation, Curettage, and Hysteroscopy 199
Burch Procedure 200

**CHAPTER 14**
PERIOPERATIVE ISSUES ............................. 203
Preoperative Considerations 203
Surgical Consent 204
Postoperative Orders 205
Postoperative Pain Relief 206
Postoperative Complications 208

**APPENDIXES**                                211

**APPENDIX A**
WORLD HEALTH ORGANIZATION
CLASSIFICATION OF FEMALE GENITAL
MUTILATION ................................................. 213

**APPENDIX B**
STAGING OF GYNECOLOGIC CANCERS ... 215
Vulvar Carcinoma—Surgically Staged 216
Vaginal Carcinoma—Clinically Staged 216
Cervical Carcinoma—Clinically Staged 216
Uterine Carcinoma—Surgically Staged 217
Fallopian Tube Carcinoma—Surgically Staged
  (Abbreviated) 218
Ovarian Carcinoma—Surgically Staged 218
Breast Carcinoma—Surgically Staged 218

**APPENDIX C**
DICTATIONS OF FIVE SURGERIES ............. 220
Abdominal Hysterectomy with Bilateral
  Salpingo-Oophorectomy 221
Vaginal Hysterectomy 222
Diagnostic Laparoscopy 223
Dilation and Curettage with Hysteroscopy 224
Burch Procedure with Insertion of Suprapubic
  Catheter 224
Index 227

# 1
PART

## The Gynecology Clinic

# 1

## CHAPTER

# *The Gynecologic History and Physical*

As with other medical disciplines, the best diagnostic tools for assessing gynecologic complaints are, of course, the history and physical examination. Before reviewing the patient interview and pelvic exam, let's review a brief description of female reproductive anatomy.

## GYNECOLOGIC ANATOMY

The most visible of the female genitalia is the pubic hair, which rests on skin overlying fatty tissue in front of the pubic bone (Fig. 1–1). The hair, skin, and underlying tissue together are called the mons pubis. The entire region between the thighs (in both men and women) is known as the perineum; in women, it is referred to more specifically as the vulva. The next structures, between the thighs, are two thick folds of skin called the labia majora. If they are separated, several structures are revealed. The small bump of skin closest to the front is the clitoris. It is partially covered by folds of skin known as the hood of the clitoris. Moving backward, the next structure is the urethral meatus. Farther back is the vaginal opening or introitus, which is par-

3

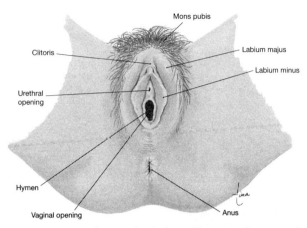

**Figure 1–1.** Female genitalia. (Adapted from Scanlon, VC and Sanders, T: Essentials of Anatomy and Physiology, ed 2. F. A. Davis, 1995, p 467, with permission.)

tially covered by folds of skin on either side, called the labia minora.

The vaginal opening may be partly or completely blocked by thin tissue known as the hymen. In women who have given birth, the hymen is often difficult to see. A few inches behind the vagina is the anus. The region between the vagina and the anus is called the posterior fourchette. The important structures of the perineum, from front to back, are the clitoris, urethra, vagina, and anus.

The vagina, a muscular tube several inches long, is normally collapsed. Bath water does not enter to any significant degree. When a woman is standing, the vagina slants backward at a 45-degree angle and runs in front of and parallel to the rectum (Fig. 1–2). The cervix, which indents the top front wall of the vagina, is a smooth, firm structure, similar in consistency to the nose. It has a small opening in its center known as the os, which is the beginning of the cervical canal. This opening is approximately the diameter of a cotton swab—slightly smaller in nulliparous women and slightly larger in parous women.

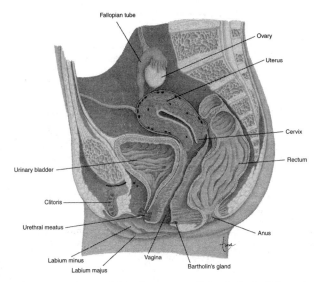

**Figure 1–2.** Internal female anatomy (lateral view). (Adapted from Scanlon, VC and Sanders, T: Understanding Human Structure and Function. F. A. Davis, Philadelphia, 1997, p 361, with permission.)

The cervix is inseparable from the womb, or uterus. The adult uterus itself is roughly half the size of a woman's fist. It lies just in front of and above the vagina and behind the bladder.

The fallopian tubes, or oviducts, are thinner than a man's little finger but are up to 4 inches long. They are attached to either side of the uterus at the upper outer portion (Fig. 1–3). The free end of each fallopian tube has thin, fingerlike projections called fimbria. Contrary to popular belief, the fallopian tubes are not physically attached to the ovary but end nearby, usually within 5 or 6 mm. The ovaries are roughly 5 cm long and 2 to 3 cm in diameter. They are suspended in the pelvis by ligaments that allow them some movement. They lie very low and deep in the pelvis, just behind the uterus.

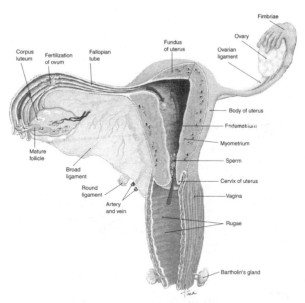

**Figure 1–3.** The female reproductive organs. (From Scanlon, VC and Sanders, T: Understanding Human Structure and Function. Philadelphia. F. A. Davis, Philadelphia, 1997, p 362, with permission.)

## GYNECOLOGIC HISTORY

As a general rule, all women between menarche and menopause should be capable of being pregnant. Women with only one sexual partner in the previous 12 months are less likely to have sexually transmitted diseases than those with multiple partners. A good history should establish the following:

1. Last menstrual period
2. Normal length of menstrual cycle (from day 1 of one cycle to day 1 of the next)
3. Number of sexual partners in previous year (usually applicable only to single women)
4. Pregnancy history
5. Current contraception method

Other questions such as age at menarche, type of sexual relations experienced, and age at first sexual intercourse should be pursued only if the questions are immediately relevant to the presenting complaint. **PEARL: Questions about the patient's symptoms provide more information if they are asked in an open-ended manner (e.g., "Where does it hurt?" rather than "Does it hurt here?").**

Abused women can present with a wide variety of complaints. Therefore, patients with symptoms that seem out of the ordinary should be asked if their partner ever hits them. It may be helpful to ask the patient if her partner has a drug or alcohol abuse problem because many physically abusive men also have substance abuse issues. When listening to patients, it helps to remember that, because much of the female reproductive anatomy is hidden, patients often have different perceptions of their bodies than do health professionals. For instance, many women say that an irritation is "inside" when they mean between the labia—an area actually outside the vagina.

## PELVIC EXAMINATION

Although women of all ages undergo this exam, it seems to provoke unusual anxiety among young women. Older women do not relish the examination, but they have a better idea of what to expect. Usually, most gynecologists also perform a general physical at least once a year. The breast examination, often considered part of a gynecologic exam, is discussed in Chapter 10, which reviews malignancies. A description of the three basic parts of the pelvic exam follows. The entire procedure is completed in 2 to 3 minutes without rushing and should not be uncomfortable.

### Inspection of the Vulva, Vagina, and Cervix

Systematically examine the vulva, starting with the clitoral area and moving downward toward the rectum. Next, gently insert a speculum into the vagina by pressing primarily against the posterior wall of the vagina, which is less sensitive than the anterior wall. Open the blades slowly and adjust them so that the cervical os is visible. A Papanicolaou (Pap) smear can be obtained at this time by placing a Cytobrush or similar swab into the cervical canal and rotating it briefly. Then place a wooden spatula in contact with the cervical portio (formerly called the portio vaginalis cervicis) and rotate it similarly. If the patient complains of a vaginal discharge, collect a sample of it and place it on a microscope slide. After obtaining the Pap smear, carefully observe the vaginal walls collapsing inward as the speculum is withdrawn, providing a final glimpse of the vaginal mucosa. The Pap slide should be smeared and fixed within seconds of obtaining the specimen because the cytologic analysis is uniquely sensitive to artifact caused by air drying. Cervical cultures for gonorrhea, chlamydia, or herpes and a vaginal smear can also be obtained at this time.

## Bimanual (Two-Handed) Exam

Place one or two fingers inside the woman's vagina and then place the other hand on her lower abdomen. In this manner, you can feel the uterus and ovaries. It takes several hundred exams to be reasonably comfortable in knowing what is normal and what is not. The size and orientation of the uterus can be described, as well as unusual lumpiness, softness, or mobility (excessive or restricted). Also make note of abnormal masses or tenderness in the adnexa (the general region of the fallopian tubes and ovaries).

## Rectal-Vaginal Exam

Place your second finger in the vagina and your third finger in the rectum while keeping your other hand in position on the lower abdomen. This position permits the detection of masses or enlarged ovaries behind the uterus. Again, the presence or absence of abnormal masses and tenderness should be noted. If desired, a sample of stool can be tested at this time for occult blood, although this test is usually confined to middle-aged and postmenopausal women.

## Recording the Exam

The proper method of recording physical findings varies among institutions. In the absence of specific instructions to the contrary, use the following notations for a normal exam:

- V, V, C (for vulva, vagina, and cervix): Normal
- Uterus: Anterior, normal size
- Adnexa, R-V (rectal-vaginal): Without abnormal masses or tenderness, heme negative (if tested)

## MAKING THE EXAM MORE BEARABLE

A pelvic examination is a significant indignity. Several steps can make it less unpleasant:

1. Before touching the patient's perineum, gently touch a less personal part of her body, such as a knee or a thigh. This gives the patient a moment to adjust to being physically examined.
2. Don't use a cold metal speculum. Some practices use plastic, disposable specula. If these are unavailable, warm the metal speculum by hand or under warm running water.
3. Separate the labia with the nondominant hand before inserting the speculum. Insert the speculum slowly; the exam will not be painful if the vaginal walls are separated slowly.
4. Tell the patient what will be done before doing it. (For instance, say, "I am now going to look inside the vagina and take a Pap smear," or "I am placing a finger in your rectum; this will be a little uncomfortable.")
5. **PEARL: It is typically unproductive to tell the patient to relax. This is a universal admonition that health care professionals give their patients who are about to undergo some invasion of their privacy that is usually also painful. No one could possibly relax under such circumstances, but patients can do things to facilitate the exam or procedure.** In the case of the pelvic exam, simply ask the patient to let her knees "flop out to either side." For patients who simply cannot cooperate, it is sometimes helpful to hold a hand out to the

side and have the patient hit the hand with her knee and then repeat the process on the other side.

6. Tell the patient what was found after the exam. In most cases, the results of the exam are normal, and telling the patient about them provides some psychological compensation for the intrusion into her personal space.

7. Finally, talk to the patient throughout the exam about nonmedical subjects such as her family, work, or news events. This technique requires skill and experience, but the intent is to distract the patient from the examination. Given the chance, most patients are quite happy to talk about something else, and it can greatly reduce the self-consciousness and anxiety surrounding the visit.

The examiner must be emotionally prepared to stop the exam at any point if it proves too uncomfortable. Patients who cannot tolerate a pelvic exam can receive oral sedation before a return visit or may even be examined under anesthesia. With patience and gentleness, however, sedation is rarely necessary.

*CONTROVERSY: There is hardly ever a circumstance in which the information revealed by an exam is so valuable that the patient should have to experience significant pain. Ironically, when the patient believes that the exam will be stopped immediately at her request, she will frequently cooperate more fully; she feels that she has a modicum of control*

## FEMALE CIRCUMCISION

A practice common to some cultures in Africa has gained notoriety with the influx of African immigrants to Western countries. Although generally intended to help protect young women against lust, these procedures are often very disturbing to Western doctors and in fact are commonly referred to as female genital mutilation in Western literature. In counseling patients who have had these procedures, it is important to be nonjudgmental and to avoid the use of emotion-laden terms such as mutilation.

In the most radical form of this practice, the vaginal opening is actually sewn almost completely closed and typically needs to be surgically incised to permit childbirth (or even comfortable intercourse) when the girl marries. Appendix A gives an abridged version of the World Health Organization Classification of Female Genital Mutilation.

# 2
## CHAPTER

# *Menstruation and Abnormal Bleeding*

Concerns related to vaginal bleeding are the most common clinical problem faced by gynecologists. Being familiar with the physiology of the menstrual cycle is a prerequisite to diagnosis and treatment of abnormal bleeding.

## THE MENSTRUAL CYCLE

The purpose of the menstrual cycle is twofold: (1) to make an oocyte available for fertilization and (2) to prepare the uterus for a possible pregnancy. If pregnancy does not occur, the thickened lining of the uterus is shed in the form of menstrual bleeding and is then rebuilt during the next cycle.

A young woman's first menstrual period or menses, called menarche, usually occurs at age 12, although the time of onset may vary (see section entitled Menarche and Puberty). In early adolescence, menstrual periods are irregular for the first year or two and do not necessarily indicate when a girl first becomes fertile. She can actually ovulate and become pregnant before her first period. Conversely, full fertility does not usually occur until a young woman has been menstruating for several years. Menses cease altogether at about age 51, signaling the beginning of menopause.

The average amount of blood lost during a menstrual period is 30 mL. A loss of more than 80 mL is considered abnormal. The menstrual cycle is determined by the number of days between the first day of one cycle and the first day of the next cycle. A typical interval is 28 days, although an interval anywhere from 21 to 35 days can be considered normal. Bleeding usually lasts from 3 to 5 days, with extremes between 1 and 8 days. Many fertile, nonpregnant women who are not on hormones have at least one irregular cycle per year.

Day 1 of the menstrual cycle begins with the first day of menstrual bleeding. The cycle ends with the start of the next period. During the days of vaginal bleeding, the hormones estrogen and progesterone, secreted by the ovary, are at their lowest output level. Slowly, the amount of estrogen secreted begins to rise. At the same time, approximately 12 oocytes start to mature. As they are prepared for release, the cells around them produce fluid that collects in a cyst or follicle. The oocytes mature until the follicle containing one of them reaches an average of 18 to 25 mm in diameter and then breaks open, releasing the oocyte into the abdomen. Remaining follicles then collapse and disappear. Rarely, two oocytes might be released if two follicles become large enough simultaneously. Release of the oocyte into the abdomen is known as ovulation. The part of the menstrual cycle that begins with the first day of vaginal bleeding and ends with ovulation is known as the follicular phase.

At the time of ovulation, the oocyte more or less floats into the end of the fallopian tube, where mild contractions of the tube, along with the motions of the tiny hairs lining it, move the egg toward the uterus. If fertilization is to take place, it usually occurs in the outer portion of the tube, close to the ovary. It is thought that the oocyte has the ability to be fertilized for only 48 hours. Fertilized or not, it takes a day or two to traverse the tube. If a pregnancy has not occurred, the egg dissolves in the uterus.

Some women can actually tell when they ovulate because they feel a pain on one side of the pelvis. The pain, known as mittelschmerz, is usually only a mild discomfort for several hours. Rarely, the pain can be so severe that it may at first appear to be a serious problem such as appendicitis.

Women occasionally have some vaginal spotting at the time of ovulation. If ovulation has been delayed for some reason, couples might mistake this bleeding as the beginning of the menses and have unprotected intercourse, thinking that this is a "safe" time.

What happens to the cells that surrounded the oocyte after it has been released from the ovary? They rapidly coalesce to form a structure within the ovary known as the corpus luteum, which produces progesterone for 12 to 14 days. After ovulation, the progesterone secreted by the ovary helps to stabilize the uterine lining and prepare it for a possible pregnancy. In the absence of conception, the corpus luteum stops producing progesterone after 14 days, and the lining of the uterus is promptly shed. If fertilization takes place, the corpus luteum will produce progesterone steadily for several weeks until the placenta can take over the job.

The portion of the menstrual cycle that starts with ovulation and ends with the beginning of the next period is logically called the luteal phase. The luteal phase almost always lasts 12 to 14 days. The follicular phase, on the other hand, varies in length from woman to woman.

The menstrual cycle is regulated by the hypothalamus, a portion of the brain that secretes pulses of gonadotropin-releasing hormone (GnRH) in varying amounts at changing frequencies (Fig. 2–1). GnRH, in turn, modulates the pattern with which the pituitary secretes two more hormones, follicle-stimulating hormone (FSH) and luteinizing hormone (LH). During the follicular phase of the cycle, FSH is secreted in steadily increasing amounts. This causes the ovarian follicles to develop and produce larger amounts of estrogen. When the amount of circulating estrogen reaches a specific level over a certain period, the pituitary then secretes a large burst of LH, called the LH surge. This surge causes ovulation to occur and the corpus luteum to form.

The relationships among the hypothalamus, pituitary, ovary, and uterus provide clues as to why two women may begin menstruating at the same time after several months of living together in the same college dorm and why women exposed to sudden psychological or physical stresses often have missed or delayed periods. Female athletes frequently stop menstruating alto-

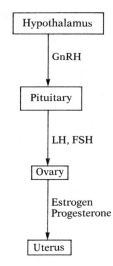

**Figure 2–1.** The link between brain and uterus.

gether because hormonal and neurologic alterations disrupt the hypothalamic release of GnRH.

Home ovulation detection kits work because of the biology of hormone secretion. These tests measure the amount of LH in the urine and turn positive with the LH surge, indicating that ovulation is about to occur.

## MENARCHE AND PUBERTY

Timing information for key events in female puberty varies slightly among different investigators. Part of this disparity can be attributed to the fact that in Western nations, the average age of first menses has decreased by 3 to 4 months per decade for the past 100 years. It is thought that better nutrition and less disease have led to this earlier onset of puberty.

In most girls, the first sign of puberty is the beginning of breast development (Table 2–1). This is followed by the appearance of pubic hair and then the growth spurt, during which axillary hair often appears. Menarche (first menses) is a relatively late occurrence in this chain of events.

**Table 2–1. CHRONOLOGIC ORDER OF
FEMALE PUBERTAL EVENTS**

Breast budding
Pubic hair development
Axillary hair
Growth spurt
First menstrual period

Breast development begins on average at age 10½ years of age, and menarche typically occurs about 2 years later. It is important to realize that both the age at which all the previously mentioned physical changes take place and the order in which they occur are highly variable. For instance, initial breast budding normally occurs anywhere between ages 8 and 13, and sometimes a little earlier or later. The first menstrual period normally occurs between ages 9 and 16, although the average age in the United States is 12. The entire process from the first signs of puberty to first menses can normally take from 1½ to 8 years.

The average height of girls in the United States at the time of menarche is roughly 5 feet, 2 inches, and their average weight is 105 pounds. As girls mature, their ratio of fat to body water increases. By the time of their first period, their weight is characteristically 27% fat and 52% water.

Exercise and weight have a strong impact on the timing of events. Girls weighing 20% to 30% more than their ideal weight tend to have an earlier menarche than they might have had otherwise; girls heavier than this tend to have a later menarche. Girls who are lighter than they should be or who exercise regularly and strenuously during early adolescence also tend to have menarche at a later age. In particular, ballet dancers, swimmers, and runners have an average age of menarche of 15. Young women with anorexia nervosa similarly have a delay in or even an absence of the start of periods. Barring heavy exercise regimens or extremes in weight, the age of menarche tends to be influenced by the mother's menstrual history.

To add to a young girl's concerns, the growth of various parts of her body proceeds at different rates. The feet and hands begin a period of accelerated growth before the lower legs and forearms, which, in turn, have a growth spurt that precedes that of the thighs and upper arms. Thus, young teenagers may feel that they have "big feet" that are out of proportion to the rest of their body. Although this may actually be true, it is a short-lived problem.

In 1960, Marshall and Tanner gave a detailed description of the stages of breast and pubic hair growth (Table 2–2). Despite such apparently precise classifications, there is much variation in the final appearance of both the breast tissue and the pubic hair. Asian women tend to have less body hair, whereas Mediterranean women tend to have more body hair. About one-fourth of all women have some hair on their abdomen, particularly in the middle.

What about abnormalities in puberty? A physician should be consulted if the first signs of puberty begin before age 7 or do not appear by age 13. Further, at the time of menarche, a physician should be consulted if a young woman is beset with disabling cramps or other

### Table 2–2. MARSHALL AND TANNER'S CLASSIFICATION OF BREAST AND PUBIC HAIR GROWTH

| Stage | Breast | Pubic Hair |
|-------|--------|------------|
| 1 | Prepubertal | No hair |
| 2 | Breast buds | Wisps of hair on labia |
| 3 | Further breast enlargement | Hair on mons pubis in midline |
| 4 | Areola forms distinct mound on breast | Hair spreads outward |
| 5 | Breast fills out—areola forms single contour with breast | Hair forms inverse triangle, reaching inner thighs |

discomforts, because very effective and easily tolerated medications are available to relieve these problems.

## FEMININE HYGIENE

Most gynecologic texts have very little information on feminine hygiene products and douching. This seems strange because women frequently discuss these topics with health professionals. In active women who bathe daily, the vagina and vulva are usually odorless. One would not think so, however, from the proliferation of advertisements in the American media for scented feminine hygiene products. Scents and sprays are almost never necessary for good hygiene, and they frequently cause allergic reactions and skin irritations. Good hygiene begins with drying off thoroughly after a bath or shower and wearing undergarments made of fabric that "breathes" (such as cotton) and clothes that are not too tight.

Young girls should be taught to wipe the perineum from front to back after urinating or defecating. A good hygiene practice in itself, this was thought to be important in preventing urinary tract infections. It now appears that the issue is more complex, but this technique remains a good recommendation.

Many people believe that sex during the menstrual period is inherently harmful and increases the risk of infection. Although some sexually transmitted diseases do seem to thrive during the menses, the responsible organisms would probably have been spread by sex even at a different time in the cycle. There is no compelling health reason to avoid sex during menses. More of a problem for some is the extreme messiness of sexual contact during the days of heavy flow. A diaphragm can make sex more hygienic during the period. It should be inserted an hour or so before sex and removed immediately afterward if the period is entirely normal and contraception is not a concern.

### Sanitary Napkins and Tampons

Sanitary napkins are easier to use than tampons and cannot be dismissed. Tampons offer an advantage, particularly for athletes, because they are invisible from the outside. Also, by preventing menstrual blood from reaching air, they eliminate the odor sometimes associated with sanitary napkins. The insertion of tampons does not cause a woman to lose her virginity, although tampons can tear a hymen that has a particularly small opening. It is not uncommon for tampons to be inserted and then forgotten. Although this practice is definitely not recommended, it is still very improbable that toxic shock syndrome will develop. The most likely outcome of forgetting to remove a tampon is the development of a malodorous discharge that ceases when the tampon is removed (see Chapter 3).

Tampons are primarily composed of cotton and polyacrylic rayon. The difference in absorbency among various products depends on their precise composition. In general, a tampon should not be left in place for more than 12 hours, and it is prudent to change them more frequently.

The addition of deodorants to both napkins and tampons can cause allergic reactions in some women. This is manifested by redness and itching of the vulva. The symptoms generally become worse with repeated exposure to the same product.

## Douches

Whether or not it is necessary to douche has long been the subject of controversy. Douching does not seem to be necessary for good health, but many women feel cleaner and fresher afterward and there is probably no harm in doing it once a week or so (not daily). Medicated and scented products are not only expensive but also can cause contact dermatitis. A preferable solution for douching consists of 1 tbsp of white vinegar or 2 tsp of salt per quart of water. The technique of douching is rather easy, although it is important that the douche bag not be suspended too high. Forcing fluid under excessive pressure can push vaginal bacteria into the normally sterile uterus and fallopian tubes. While the woman lies flat, she should insert the douche nozzle into the vagina using gentle, steady pressure until resistance from the back wall is encountered. With one hand she should pinch the labia closed around the douche nozzle and open the valve until a mild fullness is felt in the vagina. The fluid should be allowed to escape and the process repeated until the reservoir bag is empty. Most douche kits come with diagrams and further instructions.

Douching should not be done in the first few days of the menstrual cycle, when the cervix is somewhat more dilated and backflow of fluid into the uterus would theoretically be easier. Enema equipment should not be used for douching because it would introduce fecal material directly into the vagina.

## DYSMENORRHEA

Painful menstruation is classified as either primary or secondary dysmenorrhea. Primary dysmenorrhea is thought to be physiologic in origin and is defined as painful periods with an onset within a few years of menarche. It is thought to be associated with increased prostaglandin production during ovulatory cycles. For this reason, young teens, who tend to be anovulatory for the first few years after menarche, may eventually develop dysmenorrhea when they start to ovulate. Secondary dysmenorrhea is painful menstruation that starts well after ovulatory cycles have begun, typically after age 20. It suggests underlying pathology, but this is often speculative. **PEARL: One classic disease process that causes secondary dysmenorrhea is endometriosis, but this malady should not be diagnosed on the basis of symptoms alone.**

Treatment of dysmenorrhea, whether primary or secondary, typically consists of inhibiting ovulation through hormonal contraceptives or inhibiting the production of prostaglandins through the use of antiprostaglandins. Oral contraceptives, medroxyprogesterone (Depo-Provera), and levonorgestrel implants (Norplant) are all highly effective in reducing the severity of dysmenorrhea. The nonsteroidal antiinflammatory agents that inhibit prostaglandin production include two over-the-counter agents, ibuprofen (e.g., Advil) and naproxen sodium (e.g., Aleve).

Ibuprofen dosage is two 200-mg tablets every 4 hours, and naproxen dosage is 2 tablets orally to start and then one 220-mg tablet every 8 hours. These drugs can cause gastric ulcers with overuse. Surgical treatment of dysmenorrhea, which may include destruction of the medial aspects of the uterosacral ligaments or a presacral neurectomy, is almost never necessary.

## INFREQUENT MENSTRUATION

An abnormally long interval between menstrual periods may be defined as a cycle longer than 35 days; most ovulatory cycles result in withdrawal bleeding within this time span. The single most common (and important) cause of infrequent and delayed menses is pregnancy, and urine pregnancy tests should be performed if there is any suspicion of pregnancy (usually there is). The next most common reason for infrequent menstruation is anovulation (that is, some disruption in the hypothalamus has thrown off the pituitary secretion of gonadotropins, which, in turn, disrupts ovulation).

**PEARL: In women with persistently long cycles (longer than 5 weeks), prolactin and thyroid function tests should be performed because these endocrine disorders can result in anovulatory cycles (Fig. 2–2).** During the same office visit, any one of several progestins (Table 2–3) can be prescribed to induce withdrawal bleeding. If estrogen priming of the endometrium has been sufficient, a menstrual period should occur within 7 days of finishing the medication. Patients are often confused on this point and mistakenly believe that they should experience bleeding while taking the medication.

Patients who have normal prolactin and thyroid-stimulating hormone (TSH) levels, and in whom withdrawal bleeding follows a course of progestins, may be given oral contraceptive pills, or they may choose to take a progestin regularly. Women who have years of anovulatory cycles with unopposed estrogen production have an increased risk of endometrial cancer. In women who fail to have any bleeding following progestin withdrawal, LH and FSH levels should be assessed several weeks later. **PEARL: High LH and FSH lev-**

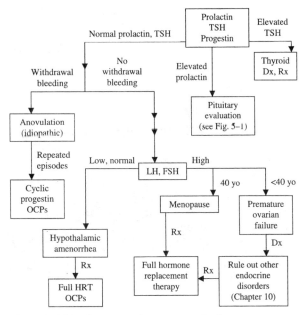

**Figure 2–2.** Evaluation and treatment of infrequent menstruation. Pregnancy should always be ruled out *first*. HRT = hormome replacement therapy; OCP = oral contraceptive pill; TSH = thyroid-stimulating hormone.

els in women younger than 40 years of age suggest premature ovarian failure (see Chapter 8); low levels at any age suggest hypothalamic dysfunction. Women with low levels of LH and FSH should be urged to use oral contraceptive pills or start hormone replacement therapy because the ovary is not producing enough estrogen to prime the uterus to respond to progestin withdrawal. Without supplemental hormones, these women are at greater risk for heart disease and osteoporosis. Hypothalamic anovulation is strongly associated with significant stress (e.g., incarceration, divorce, death of a close family member), eating disorders, and heavy exercise (e.g., the equivalent of running 20 miles per week or more).

**Table 2–3. PROGESTINS THAT CAN
BE USED TO INDUCE
WITHDRAWAL BLEEDING**

| Agent | Dose | Days | Comments |
|---|---|---|---|
| Provera (medroxy-progesterone acetate) | 10-mg tablets | 5 or 10 days | Longer treatment more effective |
| Prometrium | 400 mg (available in 100-mg tablets) | 12 days | Avoid in those with peanut allergies. Dizziness, drowsiness reduced with bedtime dosing |
| Crinone (progesterone gel) | 0.4% (45 mg) 0.8% (90 mg) | Apply with vaginal applicator for 6 days | Higher dose more effective |

## POLYCYSTIC OVARIAN SYNDROME (PCOS)

Some women with infrequent periods are also overweight and have excess body or facial hair. This clinically evident triad of hirsutism, obesity, and infrequent menses is known as polycystic ovarian syndrome (PCOS), which was first described by Stein and Leventhal in the 1930s. Our understanding of this disorder has significantly changed in the last few decades. Originally, the finding of ovaries with multiple cysts was viewed as confirmation of the diagnosis. Now, however, it is recognized that PCOS has a variety of endocrine causes and actually represents the end result of widely varying pathologic processes. The diagnosis today still relies on the clinical presentation and can be further suggested by laboratory evidence such as increased amounts of androgen or an LH-to-FSH ratio of 3:1 or greater. **PEARL: To the confusion of many, ultrasound plays no role in the diagnosis of PCOS, and the presence or**

**absence of cysts on the ovaries is not relevant in following the course of the disease.**

Because PCOS is highly variable, the treatment depends on specific patient complaints. In general, the oral contraceptive pill is very effective in both regulating menses and reducing hirsutism because it prevents ovarian production of androgen, which is often increased in these patients. Typically, the hirsutism persists for a few months before improvement is seen. For those who wish to conceive, ovulation induction is in order, usually beginning with clomiphene citrate and then moving to gonadotropins, if necessary. There is no special treatment for obesity associated with this syndrome other than diet and exercise. Weight loss among these patients does not ensure a resumption of normal menses or a reduction in hirsutism.

## EXCESSIVE BLEEDING

Abnormal, excessive bleeding should be defined as bleeding episodes that occur more frequently than 21 days apart (day 1 to day 1 of each episode) or bleeding episodes that last longer than 7 consecutive days. In women who are in their reproductive years, it is critical to exclude pregnancy as a possibility with an office urine test. In terms of diagnosing and treating frequent bleeding episodes, it is usually more productive to wait until at least two such episodes have occurred in a 6- to 12-month period before proceeding with a workup. Many women experience at least one early or heavy period per year, and this is usually a self-limited problem.

**PEARL: Even though the absorbency of napkins and tampons is listed on the box, it is remarkably difficult to obtain an accurate estimate of menstrual blood loss even by taking a careful history. Whenever there is a question of excessive menstrual bleeding, it is always wise to back up clinical estimates with a hematocrit.** Check the hemoglobin level at least once in any woman who complains of frequent or heavy bleeding, because history taking is often a very unreliable predictor of who is anemic. An occasional ambulatory patient presents with a hematocrit of 15%. Patients with hematocrits less than 30% should be more aggressively evaluated with some sort of endometrial sampling early in the workup, regardless of the patients' age. A coagulation profile should also be considered for anyone who is anemic, although bleeding disorders remain uncommon in this group.

**PEARL: As a rule, there are three common causes of frequent bleeding: anovulation, benign uterine abnormalities such as polyps or submucous myomas, and endometrial hyperplasia or malignancy.** Because endometrial cancer is rare in women younger than age 40, the approach for younger women is somewhat different than for those 40 years and older and among those who do not have significant anemia (Fig. 2–3).

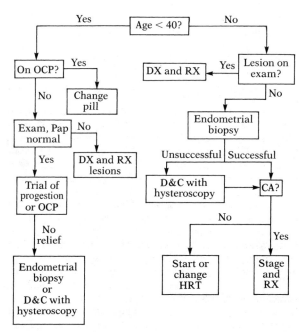

**Figure 2–3.** Evaluation and treatment of frequent bleeding. HRT = hormone replacement therapy; OCP = oral contraceptive pill; D&C = dilation and curettage.

**CONTROVERSY: Women younger than age 40 are usually given a trial of oral contraceptives if their exam is normal. An alternative is 10 mg of Provera or 200 mg of Prometrium (daily for day 16 through day 25 of each month), although this is usually less effective.**

Women older than 40 who have two episodes of frequent or prolonged bleeding should receive an endometrial biopsy before any treatment, as should women who have significant anemia or obvious risk factors for endometrial cancer, such as a long history of infrequent menses.

For women younger than 40 who do not respond to several months of oral contraceptives, some sort of histologic sampling of the uterus should be attempted. Submucous myomas and endometrial polyps are detected by an office biopsy. For continued bleeding along with a normal pathology report, there are two methods for assessing the uterine cavity, hysteroscopy and hysterosonogram. Hysteroscopy refers to placing a viewing device through the cervical canal and directly into the uterus. It can be done in the office with specialized equipment or in conjunction with a dilation and curettage (D&C) on an outpatient basis under sedation. An alternative to hysteroscopy for finding intrauterine lesions is the hysterosonogram, in which a transvaginal ultrasound is performed while the uterine cavity is distended with sterile water, making anatomic abnormalities more visible. A limitation of this technique is that it does not provide tissue for histologic examination. With liberal use of endometrial biopsy in the office to exclude malignancy, relatively few women should need a D&C and hysteroscopy under sedation or general anesthesia.

Occasionally, a patient presents with true vaginal hemorrhage, in which she is saturating more than two pads an hour for several hours in a row and is experiencing a drop in her blood count over a few hours or days. **PEARL: Vaginal hemorrhage can be controlled by administering intravenous conjugated estrogen (Premarin), 25 mg every 6 hours for up to three doses.** Typically, bleeding slows within 12 to 18 hours of the first dose of Premarin. At some point these patients should have an endometrial biopsy or a D&C with hysteroscopy to exclude endometrial cancer. Once the bleeding is controlled, the patient should be continued on Premarin, 2.5 mg four times a day for 21 days, with the addition of Provera (medroxyprogesterone) 10 mg daily for the last 5 days. She should be warned to expect a heavy but self-limited period within 7 days of stopping the hormones. After the bleeding has been controlled, the patient may need further workup to exclude benign anatomic abnormalities.

## FIRST-TRIMESTER BLEEDING

### Miscarriage

One of the leading causes of irregular bleeding in women under the age of 50 is, of course, pregnancy. Perhaps one third of women bleed in the first trimester of pregnancy, and roughly half of these go on to miscarry. **PEARL: A note on terminology: Patients who want the pregnancy find it very distressing to hear the term abortion used to describe their condition.** Bleeding without cervical dilatation is referred to as a *threatened* miscarriage. If the cervix is dilated but no tissue has passed, the diagnosis is known as *inevitable* miscarriage. If a nonviable pregnancy has not been expelled for 4 weeks or more, the situation is termed a *missed* miscarriage. Patients who pass some but not all of the pregnancy tissue have had an *incomplete* miscarriage. Many, however, pass the tissue completely, in which case they have had a *complete* miscarriage. It is sometimes hard to differentiate among the types of miscarriage, even when the patient has saved the tissue. She will almost always continue to have daily bleeding after passing tissue if significant tissue remains. Menses typically return 4 to 8 weeks after a miscarriage.

Women who are destined to miscarry in the first trimester usually experience several hours of extremely heavy bleeding with very painful cramps, although the experience can be highly variable. When a demonstrable embryo is visible on ultrasound, these women typically experience at least some discomfort, and they can be offered a suction curettage either during the process or before, if nonviability has been established. It is important to be sure that Rh-negative women who miscarry receive Rh immune globulin (RhoGAM or the like) at the time of tissue passage. Women who have miscarried (approximately 20% of all pregnancies) are not at significantly increased risk for miscarriage in the subsequent pregnancy. Many first-trimester miscarriages are associated with chromosome abnormalities, although often no cause for the pregnancy loss can be established, and karyotypes of embryonic tissue are not routinely sought.

## Ectopic Pregnancy

**PEARL: Evaluation of a woman who is bleeding in the first trimester of pregnancy typically includes three tests: human chorionic gonadotropin (hCG) levels, progesterone level, and ultrasound (Table 2–4).** This combination of tests usually can provide a good estimate of the likelihood that the patient has an ectopic pregnancy. A suction curettage can be helpful in the diagnosis if a question remains. If chorionic villi are not obtained at the time of the procedure, or if hCG levels do not fall by at least 15% afterward, an ectopic pregnancy may be diagnosed without the need for direct visualization of the fallopian tubes via laparoscopy.

### Table 2–4. EVALUATION OF FIRST TRIMESTER BLEEDING

1. **Human chorionic gonadotropin (hCG) levels,** 2 days apart (labs can report hCGs using either the First or Second International Reference Preparation.)
   *Viable pregnancy:* levels double
   *Nonviable pregnancy:* levels plateauing or falling

2. **Progesterone level**
   *>25 ng/mL:* ectopic pregnancy highly unlikely
   *<5 ng/mL:* pregnancy not viable

3. **Transvaginal ultrasound**
   *Viable pregnancy:* embryonic heartbeat with hCG >2000 IU. (The numerical cut-off at which heartbeat should be seen varies among institutions.)

**PEARL: Once an ectopic pregnancy has been diagnosed (in a stable patient), the trend in treatment has been away from surgery and toward methotrexate.** The issues surrounding medical management include the dosing regimen of methotrexate and perhaps the placement of the drug (intramuscular versus directly into the ectopic pregnancy). Protocols still vary widely among institutions. Patients who are hemodynamically unstable or in considerable pain still require surgical removal of the pregnancy via either linear salpingostomy (incision into the tube) or partial salpingectomy (removal of a portion of the tube).

*CONTROVERSY: For those with significant internal bleeding from an ectopic pregnancy, laparotomy is often preferred, though occasionally laparoscopy is attempted.*

Whether medical or surgical treatment is used, the rate of recurrent ectopic pregnancy is about 10%.

# 3

# *Contraception*

Contraceptive choices have remained somewhat static over the past several decades, partly because of low research funding priority. The main choices for women are still hormonal contraception, the intrauterine device (IUD), barrier methods, and sterilization.

## THE COMBINATION ORAL CONTRACEPTIVE PILL

The synthetic hormones in the combination pill resemble estrogen and progesterone. By introducing them into the body in steady, significant amounts, the pill prevents the pituitary from secreting luteinizing hormone (LH) and follicle-stimulating hormone (FSH) through feedback regulation. **PEARL: Because LH and FSH are not secreted, the follicles never develop sufficiently to cause an egg to be released, so the woman who takes the pill is infertile.** This effect is only temporary; when the pill is stopped, ovulation resumes. Although lower-dose pills do not always prevent ovulation, they may still prevent pregnancy. Oral contraceptives appear to have additional effects such as thickening the cervical mucus, thereby denying the sperm access to the uterus and fallopian tubes.

An important practical point is that, as a rule, women taking oral contraceptives do not develop significant follicular cysts because they do not ovulate. This means that conditions such as mittelschmerz or ruptured cyst are unlikely in these patients. Although the pill does not prevent the development of benign ovarian tumors, these types of tumors are relatively uncommon.

## Hormonal Structure of the Pill

Two estrogens and seven progestins are commonly used in oral contraceptives (Figs. 3–1 and 3–2). One of the estrogens, mestranol, is somewhat less potent than the other estrogen, ethinyl estradiol. Despite drug company protest to the contrary, the different progestins have largely the same biologic effect, although the two progestational agents most recently introduced into the U.S. market, norgestimate and desogestrel, may be somewhat less androgenic.

## Choosing a Pill to Prescribe

In general, prescribe a low-dose oral contraceptive pill. This is defined as a pill containing 35 μg or less of estrogen. With increasing attention focused on the cost of medical care, it is also probably a good idea to permit substitution and encourage the patient to buy the cheapest brand. Ortho-Novum 1/35 probably has the most competition, and the price difference between the cheapest generic pill and branded pills can be more than double ($120 versus $240 per 12 cycles). Other for-

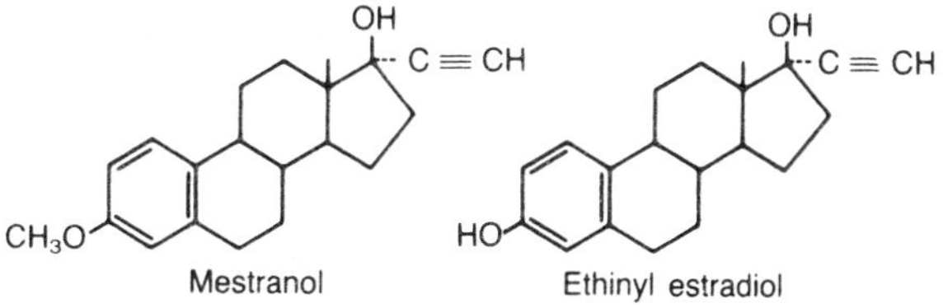

**Figure 3–1.** Synthetic estrogens used in oral contraceptives. (From Mishell, DR Jr. and Davajan, V [eds]: Infertility, Contraception, and Reproductive Endocrinology, ed. 2. Medical Economics Books, Oradell, NJ, p. 595. Reprinted with permission of Blackwell Scientific Publications, Inc.)

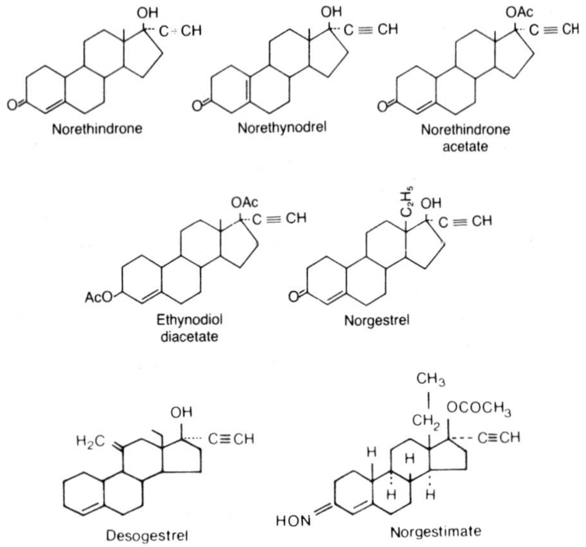

**Figure 3–2.** Synthetic progestins used in oral contraceptives. (From Mishell, DR Jr. and Davajan, V [eds]: Infertility, Contraception, and Reproductive Endocrinology, ed. 2. Medical Economics Books, Oradell, NJ, p. 594. Reprinted with permission of Blackwell Scientific Publications, Inc.) The structures of desogestrel and norgestimate were provided by Ortho-McNeil Pharmaceutical Company.

mulations also have more than one manufacturer. Examples of identical formulations include Desogen and Ortho-Cept, Triphasil and Tri-Levlen, Levlen and Nordette, and Ortho-Novum 1/35 and Norinyl 1/35. The pill generally costs less when brand competition exists than when it does not.

Table 3–1 lists more than two dozen commonly prescribed oral contraceptives. The table is organized by type of progestin; all the pills listed use ethinyl estradiol (40 μg or less) as the estrogen. In the 1990s, it is rarely necessary to use a 50-μg estrogen pill. Because the progestational agents vary in potency and biologic effect, one should not directly compare total monthly dose of progestin among different agents.

**Table 3–1. COMPOSITION OF ORAL CONTRACEPTIVES**

| Brand Name/Manufacturer | Does of Ethinyl Estradiol (μg) | Progestin Type | Daily Progestin Dose (mg) | Total Monthly Estrogen (μg)/ Progestin (mg) |
|---|---|---|---|---|
| Brevicon (Syntex) | 35 | Norethindrone | 0.5 | 735/10.5 |
| Loestrin 1.5/30 (Parke-Davis) | 30 | Norethindrone | 1.5 | 630/31.5 |
| Loestrin 1/20 (Parke-Davis) | 20 | Norethindrone | 1.0 | 420/21 |
| Modicon (Ortho) | 35 | Norethindrone | 0.5 | 735/10.5 |
| Norinyl 1+35 (Syntex) | 35 | Norethindrone | 1.0 | 735/21 |
| Ortho-Novum 1/35 (Ortho) | 35 | Norethindrone | 1.0 | 735/21 |
| Necon (Watson) | 35 | Norethindrone | 1.0 | 735/21 |
| Ortho-Novum 10/11 (Ortho) | 35 | Norethindrone | 0.5 (10 days) 1.0 (11 days) | 735/16 |
| Ortho-Novum 7/7/7 (Ortho) | 35 | Norethindrone | 0.5 (7 days) 0.75 (7 days) 1.0 (7 days) | 735/15.75 |

*Continued on following page*

**Table 3–1.** *Continued*

| Brand Name/Manufacturer | Does of Ethinyl Estradiol (µg) | Progestin Type | Daily Progestin Dose (mg) | Total Monthly Estrogen (µg)/ Progestin (mg) |
|---|---|---|---|---|
| Ovcon 35 (Mead-Johnson) | 35 | Norethindrone | 0.4 | 735/8.4 |
| Estrostep (Parke-Davis) | 20 (5 days) 30 (7 days) 35 (9 days) | Norethrindrone | 1.0 | 625/21 |
| Alesse (Wyeth-Ayerst) | 20 | Levonorgestrel | 0.10 | 420/2.10 |
| Levlen (Berlex) | 30 | Levonorgestrel | 0.15 | 630/3.15 |
| Nordette (Wyeth-Ayerst) | 30 | Levonorgestrel | 0.15 | 630/3.15 |
| Levora (Watson) | 30 | Levonorgestrel | 0.15 | 630/3.15 |
| Tri-Levlen (Berlex) | 30 (6 days) 40 (5 days) 30 (10 days) | Levonorgestrel | 0.05 (6 days) 0.075 (5 days) 0.125 (10 days) | 680/1.925 |

| | | | | |
|---|---|---|---|---|
| Triphasil (Wyeth-Ayerst) | 30 (6 days)<br>40 (5 days)<br>30 (10 days) | Levonorgestrel | 0.05 (6 days)<br>0.075 (5 days)<br>0.125 (10 days) | 680/1.925 |
| Trivora (Watson) | 30 (6 days)<br>40 (5 days)<br>30 (10 days) | Levonorgestrel | 0.05 (6 days)<br>0.075 (5 days)<br>0.125 (10 days) | 680/1.925 |
| Lo-Ovral (Wyeth-Ayerst) | 30 | Norgestrel | 0.3 | 630/6.30 |
| Demulen 1/35 (Searle) | 35 | Ethynodial diacetate | 1.0 | 735/21 |
| Zovia (Watson) | 35 | Ethynodial diacetate | 1.0 | 735/21 |
| Mircette (Organon) | 20 (21 days)<br>10 (2 days) | Desogestrel | 1.5 | 440/3.15 |
| Desogen (Organon) | 30 | Desogestrel | 0.15 | 630/3.15 |
| Ortho-Cept (Ortho) | 30 | Desogestrel | 0.15 | 630/3.15 |
| Ortho-Cyclen (Ortho) | 35 | Norgestimate | 0.25 | 735/5.25 |
| Ortho Tri-Cyclen (Ortho) | 35 | Norgestimate | 0.18 (7 days)<br>0.215 (7 days)<br>0.25 (7 days) | 735/4.515 |

A word of caution is in order before prescribing higher-estrogen pills. Some of the manufacturers that use the designations "35" and "50" to denote the amount of estrogen in their pills use ethinyl estradiol in the lower-dose version and switch to mestranol in the higher-dose version. Norinyl (made by Syntex) and Ortho-Novum (made by Ortho) are two examples. Because mestranol is somewhat less potent than ethinyl estradiol, a switch from 35 µg to 50 µg does not have the same biologic effect for all pill brands. Also, the usual reason for changing pills is to control abnormal bleeding. Rather than increasing the estrogen dose above 35 µg, try keeping the estrogen dose the same and switching to a pill with a different progestin. Although it is generally believed that breakthrough bleeding occurs less often with levonorgestrel than with norethindrone, minimizing abnormal bleeding in a specific patient tends to be a trial-and-error process.

Ortho Cyclen and Ortho Tri-Cyclen are two newer formulations that use norgestimate as the progestin. Less androgenic than the alternatives, Ortho Tri-Cyclen is the only oral contraceptive with specific Food and Drug Administration (FDA) approval for the treatment of acne.

*CONTROVERSY: Although the less androgenic norgestimate should, in theory, be better for acne than the alternative pills, no actual side-by-side clinical trials have been performed. Some other oral contraceptives may also help acne.*

## Directions for Use

There are several correct ways to start the pill. It can be started on the first day or the fifth day of the menstrual cycle or even in the middle of the cycle (with professional supervision). Because many of the lower-dose pills come packaged as "Sunday Start," however, many physicians prefer to have patients start the pills on Sunday so that they are not confused by the differences between their instructions and those on the package. Using the recommended "Sunday Start" method, the pill should be taken on the first Sunday after the first day of a period.

In the first month of pill use, patients are adequately protected from pregnancy if they start the pill within the first 5 days of the menstrual cycle. Many health care providers continue to suggest that during the first month patients use a backup method of contraception such as the condom or sponge. This approach provides an extra measure of assurance, although it may not be absolutely necessary.

The pill should be taken at roughly the same time every day to minimize the chances of unpredictable bleeding. Circumstances may arise in which a pill is missed. Any failure to take the pill on schedule reduces its reliability in preventing pregnancy. When a single pill is missed, it should be taken as soon as possible, even if this means taking two pills on the same day. The regular schedule should be continued, and no additional contraception is needed. When two pills are missed, two pills should be taken for the next 2 days. Other contraception should be used as soon as it is recognized that two pills were missed.

Those taking the 21-day pill simply do not take the pill for 7 days between packs. During this time, most women start and finish their menstrual period. They are protected against pregnancy for the entire cycle as long as they take the pills properly. Those taking the 28-day pill continue to take pills during this fourth week, but they are "filler" pills without active hormones. Then they simply start right in on the next pack as soon as the 28 pills are gone. All types of pills come in both formulations and both deliver the same amount of active ingredients; it is simply a matter of personal preference as to which pill sequence is used. Whatever pill sequence is chosen, the next cycle should be started on time even if the start occurs during the menstrual period.

With the lower-dose (and safer) pills prescribed at present, a few women experience little or no vaginal bleeding at the end of the cycle. Although this is not a threat to their health, it may be a symptom of pregnancy. Patients should be advised to perform a home pregnancy test and then call their health care provider during regular clinic hours if they have irregular or little vaginal bleeding for 2 months in a row. With two consecutive cycles of irregular bleeding, it may be prudent to change the pill. Typically, a higher estrogen dose may be helpful, or simply changing the ratio of estrogen to progestin may be sufficient. Rather than increasing the estrogen dose, the ratio can be changed by switching to a pill with a similar amount of estrogen but a different progestin. More often than not, breakthrough bleeding is resolved through trial and error.

There is no benefit or increased safety from stopping the pill intermittently for a so-called rest period. If the woman decides to become pregnant, the pill should not be taken for 3 months before the desired time of starting pregnancy. During this 3-month period, a barrier method of contraception, such as the condom, sponge, or diaphragm, should be used. Conception immediately after stopping the pill does not pose a direct threat to the fetus, but the incidence of twins and other multiple births is increased in conceptions that occur within 3 months of stopping the pill. Also, unless regular menstruation is occurring (after the pill is stopped), the woman's due date will be less certain.

Many women do not menstruate for a number of months after stopping the pill. If 6 months elapse without menses, a workup for anovulation should be considered. The pill does not cause infertility, but a woman who is subfertile before starting the pill (even if she did not know about it) would have the same problem after it is stopped. For the few women who conceive while taking the pill, the most recent analyses do not demonstrate any teratogenic potential from the oral contraceptives.

## Safety

Using the pill for 1 year is twice as safe as carrying a pregnancy to term and giving birth. In fact, it may be more than twice as safe; several studies were unable to demonstrate any increase in mortality in women younger than the age of 35. The safety of oral contraceptives is closely related to their dose of estrogen. In general, pills with 35 μg of estrogen or less have very little metabolic effect. The safety issues of the pill can be broken down into three categories: cardiovascular disease, cerebrovascular accidents, and cancer.

### Cardiovascular Disease

The risk of cardiovascular disease (hypertension, myocardial infarction, and thromboembolic disease) is related to both pill dosage and the patient's other risk factors. **PEARL: Women older than 35 who smoke or who have substantially elevated blood pressure probably should not continue to take the pill.** Smoking, hypercholesterolemia, and age all increase the probability of adverse events. Approximately 5% of women taking higher-dose pills than commonly prescribed in current practice did experience clinically significant hypertension, but with current low-dose pills, no significant tendency toward high blood pressure has been noted. This is not to say that the pill is appropriate for those with preexisting hypertension, however. The pill does not increase the risk of myocardial infarction in women younger than age 35, regardless of smoking status. Finally, the degree of excess risk of venous thromboembolism in pill users seems to be slight, if any.

### Cerebrovascular Accidents

The general sense from recent studies of low-dose pill users is that there is no increased risk. Nonetheless, women who experience a sudden onset of severe headaches or prominent visual symptoms should probably stop taking the pill, at least temporarily, pending evaluation.

### Cancer

No consistent evidence of increased risk has been found for any cancer, including, and especially, breast cancer.

**CONTROVERSY: Although almost 40 years of data have not shown an increased risk of breast cancer, the possibility of long-term latent effects from the pill has not been completely excluded, because breast cancer usually occurs postmenopausally.**

### *Other Health Problems*

Reports focusing on higher-dose pill users did show a trend toward carbohydrate intolerance (elevated blood glucose) and increased gallbladder disease. The validity of these findings with low-dose pills is still under study, but as with all of the other side effects, metabolic changes seem to be minimal with the new formulations now in widespread use.

### *Breastfeeding*

Nursing mothers can use the pill, but it seems to reduce the quantity of breast milk. A small amount of the hormone from the pill may be transferred to the baby, but no adverse effects are discernible.

## Advantages

**PEARL: The pill has numerous advantages:**
- Most effective reversible contraceptive
- Reduced anemia
- Reduced risk of pelvic inflammatory disease among women with gonorrhea
- Reduced pain of menses in most women with painful periods
- Reduced size of follicular cysts
- Reduced risk of uterine and ovarian cancer
- Significantly reduced incidence of rheumatoid arthritis (protection lost after discontinuing the pill)

## Disadvantages

The disadvantages of the pill include the obvious need to remember to take it daily and the less obvious list of possible side effects. The four most common side effects are irregular bleeding, nausea, weight gain, and depression. As a rule, these side effects disappear after two or three cycles of use. Nausea is often decreased by taking the pill on a full stomach, and it may occur only in the first few days of each cycle.

## Cost

Combination oral contraceptive pills cost about $25 to $30 for a 1-month package. Typically, 21-day and 28-day pills do not differ in price as long as the brand is the same. Several varieties of generic pills cost between $12 and $15 per cycle. Another cost consideration is that in most practices and clinics, even healthy, nonsmoking women need to be examined at least once a year.

## THE "MORNING-AFTER" PILL

The FDA has recently approved a specific prescription formulation to serve as a post-coital contraceptive: Preven, containing 50 μg of ethinyl estradiol and 0.25 mg of levonorgestrol. **PEARL: An alternative "morning-after" regimen is simply to administer combination oral contraceptive pills containing 50 μg of ethinyl estradiol two tablets orally at a time, 12 hours apart.** The first pills must be taken within 72 hours of intercourse. They are thought to prevent implantation of the embryo on the endometrium. There are probably no significant complications to the user from one-time use. Nausea is the most common side effect. Irregular bleeding during that menstrual cycle is also common. This regimen reduces the pregnancy rate by 75% and is not known to be teratogenic for pregnancies that do occur in spite of its use.

## PROGESTIN-ONLY CONTRACEPTIVES

Progestin-only contraceptives can be given orally, intramuscularly, or even via subcutaneous implants.

### Progestin-Only Pill

The progestin-only "mini-pill" differs in two ways from the combination pill. Not only does it contain no estrogen but also the progestin content is less. Because of the lower dose and progestin-only content, some women ovulate while taking this pill. But as mentioned earlier, some investigators speculate that progestins cause a thickening in cervical mucus (denying access to the uterus), disrupt transfer of the oocyte down the fallopian tube, or even prevent an embryo from attaching to the lining of the uterus. The failure rate of the minipill is about 2 to 3 per year out of 100 regular users, in contrast to less than 1 in 100 for combination pill users. These pills can be started in the same manner as the combination pills described earlier, but they must be taken every single day, with no "rest period." Other contraceptive methods should definitely be used for the first cycle. If a single pill is missed, two can be taken the next day, but other contraception should be used for that cycle. Also, if a menstrual period does not occur for 45 days, a health care professional must be notified, because this sign may signify a pregnancy. The costs of the progestin-only pill and of the combination pill are about the same—roughly $25 to $30 per month. These pills are commonly prescribed for a year at a time.

## Progestin Injections (Depo-Provera)

The contraceptive mechanism of progestin injection is similar to that of the progestin-only pill, but the medication is absorbed slowly so that its effects can last for several months. Injections are given into the buttocks or arm every 3 months. Substantial protection is conferred for up to 6 additional weeks, so there is some flexibility in giving the injection. **PEARL: Progestin injections are extremely effective in preventing pregnancy: Among those who regularly obtain their injections, only 2 women in 1000 conceive.** This success rivals or surpasses that of combination oral contraceptive pills and is much better than that of the progestin-only pill. These injections typically cost $60 to $80, which on an annual basis is comparable to the cost of a brand-name combination pill. Depo-Provera is increasingly popular among inner-city teens, and a decrease in the pregnancy rate in this community has been attributed to its increased use.

## Progestin Implants (Norplant)

The Norplant system consists of six Silastic tubes placed just beneath the skin on the underside of one arm.

It provides 5 years of pregnancy protection and is completely reversible. It releases a synthetic progestin, called levonorgestrel, at a constant rate and prevents pregnancy in much the same way as Depo-Provera. It prevents the woman from ovulating and causes her cervical mucus to thicken somewhat, thereby making it more difficult for sperm to swim up the reproductive tract.

Norplant needs to be inserted within 7 days of the beginning of a menstrual period. Gynecologists are the only doctors who are likely to perform the procedure, but not all gynecologists perform it. The procedure can be performed right in the doctor's office. The insertion itself takes 10 to 15 minutes. Injection of the anesthetic medication beneath the skin on the underside of the arm is somewhat uncomfortable, similar to the discomfort associated with a blood draw. A small skin incision (perhaps a fourth of an inch long) is then made, and the six Silastic tubes are then pushed through a hollow tube placed just underneath the skin and deposited there (Fig. 3–3). After the procedure, one or two small Steri-Strips are placed over the insertion site and covered with gauze. The gauze should be left in place for 24 hours, after which it may be removed. The arm should be kept dry for this time. After 3 days, the Steri-Strips may be taken off. The patient should call if there is redness, pain, or pus oozing from the insertion.

Removal of Norplant is similar to its insertion but more difficult. A local anesthetic is injected, and a small incision is made close to where the incision was made for insertion. A hemostat is then used to remove each of the tubes. Because a capsule of tissue can form around

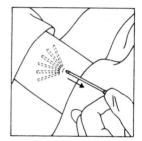

**Figure 3–3.** Norplant insertion. (Courtesy of Wyeth-Ayerst Laboratories, Philadelphia)

the implants, they can be somewhat difficult to remove. A fresh set of Norplant capsules may be inserted at the same time if desired. If removal of all the implants proves difficult at the time when the patient wishes to discontinue Norplant, a second removal attempt may be necessary 4 weeks later.

Insertion costs between $500 and $800, and the removal procedure usually costs $150 to $200. Even including both the insertion and removal costs, however, Norplant is cheaper than 5 years of brand-name oral contraceptive pills.

## Safety, Advantages, and Disadvantages of Progestin-Only Contraceptives

*CONTROVERSY: Because by definition progestin-only contraceptives do not contain estrogen, they are generally thought to entail less risk of thromboembolic events, but this reduced risk has not been conclusively established.*

It seems reasonable to believe that progestin-only contraceptives are at least as safe as combination pills. Although the "mini-pill" is slightly less effective than estrogen-progestin pills, both the injection and implant routes of administration are thought to be even more effective, with pregnancy rates measurable per 1000 women per year rather than the 100 women per year denominator used for other contraceptive measures. A big disadvantage common to all progestin-only agents is the tendency toward unpredictable bleeding or amenorrhea. Skipped periods raise the prospect of the need for pregnancy testing. As a rule, however, patients fall into a certain pattern of bleeding after the first 6 to 12 months, and pregnancy testing is necessary only when there is a significant change in an established pattern.

## THE INTRAUTERINE DEVICE

It is unclear how the IUD works. Because it can prevent pregnancy if it is inserted within several days after unprotected intercourse, many believe that the IUD prevents the fertilized egg from being implanted on the wall of the uterus. Alternatively, the IUD may interfere with sperm passage to the tubes or movement of the egg through the tubes. The medicated IUD, which contains copper or progestins, also has unresolved questions concerning its mechanism.

Effectiveness is roughly the same for all IUDs. Theoretically, they should prevent pregnancies in 99% of women for 1 year. Because the IUD can be expelled or improperly inserted, however, the actual effectiveness rate is only 95%—which is still very good.

## Insertion and Removal

Insertion of an IUD is a 5-minute office procedure. Progestin-medicated IUDs must be replaced yearly, and copper IUDs have a 10-year cycle. Other types of IUDs can remain in place indefinitely.

Because one of the chief problems with the IUD is expulsion from the uterus, the patient must check in the vagina after each menstrual cycle for the string trailing from the cervix. If she cannot feel the string, she must notify her health care provider and use a backup method of contraception. Usually the IUD is still present, and the string was simply difficult to feel.

Insertion of the device itself does not always proceed smoothly and painlessly, although it takes only a few minutes. After an examination, expose the cervical opening (tip of the uterus) with a speculum inserted into the vagina and then wash out the vagina with antiseptic solution. Then grasp the cervix with a tenaculum. At this point, the patient may feel a cramp or mild, sharp pain. Probe the uterus for size with a device known as a sound, which may also cause cramping. Then insert the IUD by placing it into a narrow, hollow barrel and then pushing it out into the uterus with a plunger once the barrel is within the womb. Once out of the barrel, the IUD expands to its normal shape (Fig. 3–4). Cut the string, or tail, of the IUD so that it protrudes from the cervix and then remove all of the instruments.

For women who have had at least one baby, the experience usually goes smoothly. IUD insertion is typi-

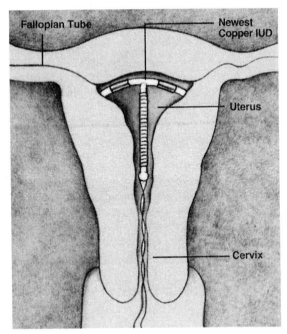

**Figure 3–4.** IUD within the uterus. (Courtesy of GynoPharma Inc., Somerville, NJ)

cally more uncomfortable for women who have not had babies, even when a smaller device is used. **PEARL: Although the IUD can be inserted at any time in the cycle, most practitioners prefer placing it toward the end of a menstrual period because the cervical canal dilates a little during menses and the insertion is less uncomfortable. This timing also offers some reassurance that the patient is not pregnant.**

Removal of an IUD is much easier. Simply grasp the string with an instrument and remove it with one tug. Fertility is restored immediately, except with the copper and progestin IUDs. Their contraceptive effect wears off in a short time.

# Safety

The safety of the IUD has been the subject of much controversy. Aside from the disadvantages, which are discussed later, there are some risks associated with insertion and two other chief safety issues: pelvic inflammatory disease (PID) and ectopic pregnancy.

The risks of insertion, including uterine perforation and improper placement, are relatively small. The risk of perforation depends directly on the skill of the person inserting the device (in the United States, usually a physician). Some have estimated the perforation rate to be as low as 1 in 2500 procedures, but it may be higher. A perforation that is recognized may or may not be a problem, because the actual damage done to the uterus usually heals rapidly without permanent consequence.

A more important issue than possible perforation is the location of the IUD after the insertion. If the IUD is not in the uterus, obviously the woman can get pregnant. Also, the IUD may cause inflammation if it is placed within the abdominal cavity. Often enough, if this event occurs, the patient remains asymptomatic, and the device can be retrieved through laparoscopy or at the time of abdominal surgery for other conditions.

The role of the IUD in increasing the risk of PID is a matter of some controversy. The risk has been most clearly demonstrated for wearers of the Dalkon shield, which has since been removed from the market. It is not entirely clear whether PID occurs more frequently in IUD wearers who are not using the Dalkon shield than in women without an IUD. Many investigators suspect that the string leading from the sterile uterus into the vagina may make it easier for uterine infection to take place.

The association of IUDs with PID is not as straightforward as it might appear. First, the overall incidence of PID in users of recently marketed IUDs is actually rather low, roughly 2.5 per 1000 women who use the device for 1 year (compared with 1 per 1000 among diaphragm users). Second, and more important, PID is not transmitted by an IUD.

**CONTROVERSY:** *Although there is concern that an IUD can increase the complication rate of gonorrhea and chlamydia, and thereby slightly increase the chances that a user will get PID, it does not increase the odds that an individual will catch gonorrhea or chlamydia. These odds are strongly linked to the number of sexual partners that a woman has over a given period. As a result, many recommend giving IUDs only to women who are in a stable marriage. This practice greatly reduces the incidence of sexually transmitted disease (STD) complications.*

With regard to ectopic (tubal) pregnancy, misunderstandings abound. It is true that the few women who do get pregnant while wearing an IUD are more likely to have a tubal pregnancy than their peers who do not use the IUD. However, the actual incidence of tubal pregnancies among IUD users is lower than among nonusers. This paradox occurs because the IUD is most effective in preventing pregnancies within the uterus, so that the few ectopic pregnancies that do occur represent a higher fraction of all pregnancies among IUD users than among nonusers.

Up to 50% of the pregnancies that occur with an IUD in place will end in miscarriage, usually in the first trimester. Although it is common practice to remove the IUD in the event of a pregnancy (because this has been shown to cut the miscarriage rate in half), miscarriage may still result. There is no evidence of an increased risk of birth defects if the pregnancy goes to term.

The most important safety concern with an IUD is a slight increase in the incidence of PID, generally a complication of gonorrhea and chlamydia. The IUD has few other significant health risks, and it is often ideal in terms of safety for married women who have finished their childbearing. The tailless IUD (without a string) is worn by millions of Chinese women, apparently with good effectiveness and safety.

## Disadvantages

The chief untoward side effect of the IUD is an increase in menstrual cramping and blood flow. This problem is minimized by confining IUD use to women who have had full-term pregnancies because they seem to be less affected.

## Cost

The cost of inserting the Paraguard IUD varies but is generally about $400 (including the $150 cost of the device itself). Because it provides protection for 10 years, its annual cost is equal to that of the least expensive contraceptive methods, barriers and spermicides.

## SPERMICIDES AND BARRIER METHODS

Most barrier methods have roughly the same effectiveness and costs, and share the same advantages and disadvantages. The arguments for their use are that they give typical users about 80% to 90% protection from pregnancy and protect against STDs to some degree. Their disadvantages are mundane but important to many couples, in that they can be messy, usually require planning in advance of each sex act, and involve direct genital manipulation before intercourse.

### Spermicides

There are several ways to disable sperm. The most widely used compound, nonylphenoxypolyethoxyethanol (nonoxynol 9), acts as a detergent that disrupts the cell membrane of the sperm. A significant side benefit of this chemical is that it destroys the surface of some bacteria, viruses, and parasites in the vagina and thus provides protection against STDs. The contraceptive effectiveness of spermicides varies significantly, from as high as 98% to as low as 70%. This wide range of effectiveness reflects the varying motivation of couples who use the substances.

Vaginal suppositories must be placed deep within the vagina and given 10 to 30 minutes to dissolve. In contrast, the creams, jellies, and foams are all active immediately after insertion into the vagina. These latter methods require that applicators, which are filled with the agent, be placed deep within the vagina and then emptied. Creams tend to be less messy than jellies. Because foams consist primarily of spermicide and gas, they are the least noticeable of all because the gas simply escapes on application. The foam container must be shaken thoroughly before use, however, and the protective effect of the foam lasts for only about 30 minutes.

It is important for the patient not to douche for at least 4 hours (some suggest 8 hours) after intercourse. With each new act of sex, additional spermicide must be placed within the vagina.

Spermicides are essentially nontoxic when used as directed. The only potential problem is an occasional allergic reaction, which is usually limited to genital irritation affecting both women and men. The irritation resolves when exposure to the spermicide is ended. As mentioned before, these chemicals tend to protect against the spread of various STDs, including gonorrhea and some viruses. Spermicides are not thought to be teratogenic for those pregnancies that result in spite of their use. The cost of spermicides is highly variable but is generally less than $1 per application.

## Condoms

The condom must be placed over the penis before any direct penis-to-vagina contact because sperm can leak out unnoticed before ejaculation. Also, care must be taken not to put the condom on too tightly. An extra ½ to 1 inch of material should be present at the tip of the penis to prevent the sperm from breaking the rubber. As soon as the man ejaculates, he should withdraw, while holding onto the condom at the base of the penis, because it is common for the sperm to spill inside the vagina if he loses his erection before withdrawing. The condom should then be removed carefully and discarded.

These simple but effective contraceptives are widely available in only one size; they are made to fit all customers. Manufacturers have introduced a large size for men who are too uncomfortable with the standard size.

Condoms are available in a variety of colors and textures, and with various lubricants.

The condom probably affords the best protection among all contraceptives against STDs, although the precise extent of this protection is unknown. The protection offered by animal-skin condoms is much less certain than for those made of latex. Many condoms can be obtained for between 30¢ and 50¢ apiece, although they can be much more expensive, depending on the specific type.

The "female" condom has recently been introduced commerically in the United States. It consists of two polyurethane rings enclosed by a thin sheath of the same material and is open at one end. It does not contain spermicide but is coated with a silicone-based lubricant. It can be inserted into the vagina up to 8 hours before intercouse. Stronger than latex condoms, it should not be used in combination with them because the two devices might adhere to each other and become dislodged. Its contraceptive efficacy is similar to the diaphragm and condom, but it may be better at preventing the spread of STDs because it partially covers the female perineum beyond the vaginal introitus.

## The Diaphragm

A diaphragm is a rubber or plastic cup that fits over the cervix. The diaphragm has two contraceptive effects. First, it serves as a barrier, preventing sperm from getting near the cervical opening. Second, the spermicide used with the diaphragm kills the few sperm that manage to get past the rim of the diaphragm.

The diaphragm must be fitted by a health care professional. As a rule, the diaphragm prescribed is the largest that will fit comfortably. It is held in place in front by resting against the pubic bone. In the back, the far wall of the vagina secures it against the cervix.

The woman should be careful not to insert the diaphragm too long before sexual intercourse takes place. It can usually be inserted up to 6 hours in advance, although some recommend an interval of no more 2 hours. After intercourse, it should be left in the vagina for 6 to 8 hours, although this recommendation is somewhat arbitrary, and 2 hours may well be long enough. The diaphragm should not usually interfere with voiding or defecation.

With every use, the diaphragm should be inspected for holes or defects, which of course would ruin its effectiveness. There is no set period after which a diaphragm must be replaced, but sometimes, replacement is required to ensure a proper fit. For example, a virgin who has a diaphragm fitted before first intercourse might have its fit rechecked several weeks afterward because the vagina might stretch somewhat. The diaphragm should also be refitted if the woman experiences significant weight changes (i.e., a gain or a loss of 20 lb or more) and after each pregnancy.

Only spermicides specifically designed for the diaphragm should be used. A variety of agents, including petroleum jelly, may actually damage the diaphragm over time. The diaphragm should not be left in the vagina continuously for more than 24 hours; this can increase the risk of toxic shock syndrome. During a menstrual period, it probably should not be left in place for more than 6 to 8 hours at a time.

Give patients the following directions for using a diaphragm:

1. Put approximately 1 tbsp of spermicide (cream or jelly) into the diaphragm, and spread it around the rim. Hold the diaphragm dome side down (as though it were a bowl).
2. To insert, pinch the diaphragm in the middle of the rim with one hand and separate the lips of the vagina with the other (Fig. 3–5). Insert it as far back into the vagina as it can go. A specially designed applicator (plastic handle) can also be used for insertion. There are three body positions in which a diaphragm can be inserted (Fig. 3–6):
   • Lying flat on the back with knees bent and flexed outward
   • Squatting
   • With one leg up on a chair or the side of the bathtub
3. Check the position of the diaphragm after insertion (Fig. 3–7). It must be resting against the pubic bone in front. This can be felt by placing a finger in the vagina and feeling the upper, forward portion. It is

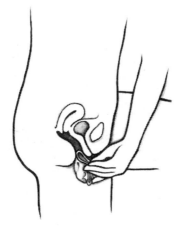

**Figure 3–5.** Diaphragm insertion. (Courtesy of Ortho-McNeil Pharmaceutical Corporation, Raritan, NJ)

important to make certain that the diaphragm is covering the cervix, which has the firmness of the tip of the nose. The cervix is deep within the vagina and is along the upper vaginal wall. A small indentation also may be felt, which is the cervical opening. When the diaphragm is in place and covering the cervix,

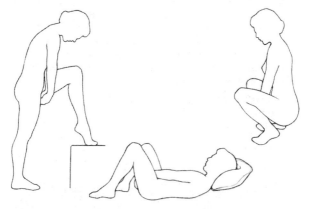

**Figure 3–6.** Diaphragm insertion positions. (Courtesy of Ortho-McNeil Pharmaceutical Corporation, Raritan, NJ)

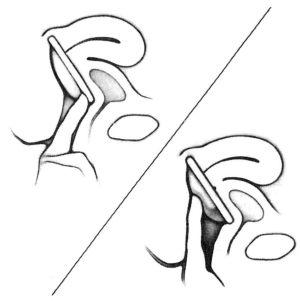

**Figure 3–7.** Checking the diaphragm position. (Courtesy of Ortho-McNeil Pharmaceutical Corporation, Raritan, NJ)

you should not be able to feel the diaphragm except with your finger.
4. To remove the diaphragm, place your finger into the vagina, reach up and forward to hook the rim, and draw the diaphragm down and out.
5. Wash the diaphragm with soap, rinse it thoroughly, and then dry. No powder or other agents are necessary during storage.

Diaphragms are extremely safe. The only health problem, which occurs infrequently, is temporary irritation caused by an allergic reaction to either the diaphragm or the spermicide. Toxic shock syndrome probably occurs in less than one per million uses, usually after the diaphragm has been left in the vagina for more than a day at a time. The diaphragm itself and the associated spermicide are thought to provide some protection against STDs, but the extent of this benefit is not known. Aside from the cost of the office appointment, the diaphragm itself costs between $30 and $50. Roughly 50¢ worth of spermicide is used with each episode of intercourse.

## The Cervical Cap

The cap is similar to the diaphragm in many respects, but it is intended to fit more precisely over the cervix. It can be left in place for up to 2 days after intercourse. It does not have the same wide availability in the United States as the diaphragm, and it requires more training in both fitting and use.

## PERIODIC ABSTINENCE

The basis of this technique (popularly known as the "rhythm method") is abstinence, generally for at least a week, in mid-cycle. However, the scientific underpinnings of this method may be changing.

*CONTROVERSY: It is widely believed that fertilization can result only from intercourse that takes place 2 days before ovulation to 1 day after it. But recent evidence suggests that fertilization may follow intercourse that occurs up to 6 days before ovulation and perhaps not even half a day after it.*

In any event, the period of abstinence is defined by estimating the time of ovulation, which can be done by plotting out cycle lengths, measuring basal body temperatures over several cycles, or following the changing consistency of cervical mucus. The efficacy of this method (around 75%) is improved by increasing the days of abstinence.

## FEMALE STERILIZATION

All operations specifically intended for female sterilization result in some type of damage to the fallopian tubes. All of the major methods of damaging the tubes appear to have roughly the same effectiveness in preventing subsequent pregnancies. These operations are simplistically grouped into one group labeled "tubal ligations," although tying the tube, as "ligation" implies, is by no means the sole method of causing tubal damage.

## Technique

Tubal ligation can be performed by the minilaparotomy or laparoscopy. The minilaparotomy involves a 2-inch incision at the level of the pubic hair line, through which the tubes are identified. The middle portion of each tube is then grasped, and a suture is placed around this isolated loop of tube. This portion of tube, which has been tied off, is then excised. The incision is sutured closed in layers, usually with dissolving sutures. This procedure typically takes 20 to 30 minutes and is performed under general anesthesia on an outpatient basis, although it can also be done with spinal anesthesia. An even more popular method of sterilization is via laparoscopy, in which the tubes are either cauterized, compressed with a clip (Hulka Clip), or rubber-banded (with the Falope ring).

The tubes can also be "tied" via a modified minilaparotomy in the immediate postpartum period (within 48 hours of birth). In this case, the 2-inch incision is made just below the umbilicus because that is the position of the enlarged uterus with its tubes immediately after birth. This procedure is often performed with spinal or epidural anesthesia, although it can also be done with general anesthesia. It often does not prolong the normal postpartum stay. The tubes can also be ligated by a vaginal approach, although this operation is somewhat more difficult and has a higher infection rate. Although its advantage is that the scar is on the inside, which results in less postoperative pain, the somewhat higher complication rate has limited its recent popularity.

These operations tend to result in minimal postoperative disability because of the small size of the incision. After laparoscopy, it is not unusual to have shoulder pain for a day or so. This occurs because the abdomen was distended, placing the diaphragm under stretch. The nerves perceiving pain from the diaphragm share a pathway with nerves from the shoulder, so that this stretching of the diaphragm is often perceived as shoulder pain. Incisional pain can be well controlled with narcotics. A typical prescription is for acetaminophen

(Tylenol codeine #3) with 30 mg of codeine, two tablets orally, every 3 to 4 hours as needed.

It is very important to use effective contraception in the months before sterilization. If a pregnancy has already implanted in the uterus, tubal ligation will do nothing to interrupt it. Also, a woman having unprotected intercourse in the days preceding sterilization has a theoretical risk of having the pregnancy settle in the damaged tube, with a resultant ectopic or tubal pregnancy. The cost of female sterilization varies depending on the medical facility used but is usually several thousand dollars. Health insurance often covers the expense.

## Effectiveness

All of the sterilization methods just described have roughly the same failure rate. After a sterilization procedure, roughly 4 out of 1000 women will become pregnant over a number of years. Although protection from pregnancy is not absolutely ensured, sterilization provides protection that is far superior even to that of the pill.

Pregnancies can occur following properly performed procedures because of the body's ability to heal itself. When a portion of tube is tied and then removed, the result is that both portions of tube scar over and separate as the suture dissolves. Once in a great while, a passageway through both scarred portions of tube can result, allowing a pregnancy to take place. The same type of process can occur with burning, clipping, or rubberbanding. After scarring has taken place, the tiny rubber band may simply drop off into the pelvis as the tube shrivels up. Rarely, a passage can develop through which the egg can be fertilized. Pregnancies have even been reported following removal of the uterus, when a passage developed from the tied-off end of the tube to the sutured-over top of the vagina.

## Safety

Risk of death from laparoscopic sterilization is thought to be in the range of 1 to 10 per 100,000 operations. Although the risk from minilaparotomy is not known, if anything, it is probably even less than that for laparoscopy. Complications include damage to abdominal organs necessitating additional, more extensive surgery to repair; hemorrhage requiring transfusion; and infections that need to be treated with antibiotics. Damage to abdominal organs is somewhat more common with laparoscopy because the procedure calls for the blind insertion of the first probe. Although the abdomen is distended at this point and the organs should be well out of the way, sometimes the probe tip does indeed cause damage. An additional complication of laparoscopy can be burns to the abdominal organs when cautery is used to burn the tube and inadvertently makes contact with adjacent structures.

The risk of anesthesia, although separate from the risk of surgery, tends to be very small. In summary, the complications from either procedure tend to be infrequent and minor. One complication of tubal ligation is not always mentioned. Although the risk of pregnancy is very small, if a pregnancy occurs, it is likely to be ectopic. **PEARL: Some studies seem to indicate that approximately 50% of all pregnancies occurring after a sterilization procedure (admittedly a small overall number) are tubal pregnancies.** Even if the tube is open, it is almost invariably damaged and has impaired function. As a result, it is not uncommon for the embryo to become trapped in the tube.

## Reversibility

Some observers estimate that approximately 10% of all women who claim never to want children again change their minds later and regret their decision for sterilization. The most frequent reason for a woman's change of heart regarding sterilization is a subsequent (and often unanticipated) divorce and remarriage. The foregoing procedures are not meant to be reversible, and they should not be requested if there is any suspicion that pregnancy may be desired at a future date. These procedures are specifically designed to cause significant, permanent damage to the tube. Although tubal ligations can be reversed approximately 70% of the time, reversal requires a major time-consuming and expensive operation.

## MALE STERILIZATION

Male sterilization, or vasectomy, involves destruction of the vas deferens, the tube that transports sperm from the testicles to the penis. After the area is prepared with antiseptic solution, local anesthetic is injected into the scrotal skin. A small incision is made in the scrotum, and the vas deferens is identified, tied off, cut, and sometimes burned. The skin is then sutured closed with dissolving stitches, and the procedure is repeated on the other side. The entire process can be performed in 15 to 30 minutes. Sterility is not immediate because sperm are stored beyond the point of damage to the vas deferens. After 10 ejaculations, the semen should be examined microscopically to be sure that it contains no sperm.

**PEARL: The death rate from vasectomy is so low that it is difficult to come up with a precise figure.** It is probably less than one out of a million operations. Although female sterilization is quite safe, the rate of major complications that result from vasectomy is significantly less. Infection and bruising can occur but are very uncommon. The operation is inherently safer than female sterilization because the abdominal cavity is never entered and local anesthesia rather than regional or general anesthesia is used.

*CONTROVERSY: A recent controversy has arisen regarding the risk of prostate cancer following vasectomy. At present, it seems that this will not prove to be a significant risk, although the issue is being more closely examined.*

Just as with female sterilization, vasectomy is not intended to be reversible. Expensive operations to restore the damaged vas deferens succeed 18% to 60% of the time.

## ABORTION

Abortion is not actually a contraceptive method because it does not prevent fertilization. However, it is included in this chapter because it is clearly a method of controlling family size, albeit a controversial one.

The evaluation for women considering an abortion includes a pelvic exam, a CBC, blood type and Rh, a urine pregnancy test, and often an ultrasound to confirm the length of pregnancy. At some point, the woman will undergo counseling in which alternatives to abortion (adoption or raising the child herself) are discussed. The mechanics of the abortion procedure are also discussed during this counseling session.

Rarely, an abortion can fail to terminate the pregnancy. **PEARL: Failure to terminate the pregnancy is most likely if the abortion is attempted too early, so abortions usually are not performed before at least 6 weeks have elapsed since the last menstrual period.** Although failure is not common, it can happen, which is one good reason for having a follow-up appointment. (Urine pregnancy tests may remain positive for as long as 2 weeks after a successful abortion.)

**PEARL: An abortion will not end an ectopic pregnancy. For this reason, the tissue obtained at the time of the abortion should always be examined microscopically to confirm the presence of chorionic villi, which, for practical purposes, excludes an ectopic pregnancy.** (Twin pregnancies with one twin in the uterus and one in the tube occur in perhaps 1 in 30,000 pregnancies.)

There are two basic types of abortion—mechanical and medically induced. Some abortion procedures use both methods.

## Dilation and Evacuation

The main mechanical method of abortion in current use is known as dilation and evacuation (D&E). With this method, the cervix is first dilated with metal rods of increasing diameter. A hollow tube, typically 8 to 12 mm in diameter, is inserted into the uterus and attaches to a vacuum machine, which then suctions out the contents of the uterus. In addition, grasping instruments are introduced into the uterus to remove any part of the pregnancy that might have been left behind. Finally, the uterine walls are curetted—gently scraped with a sharp instrument to be sure that the uterus is empty.

### *Laminaria*

**CONTROVERSY: *Although the methods vary somewhat, for many health care providers, the next step after the***

*counseling session is the insertion of laminaria, small sticks of dried seaweed that swell on exposure to moisture; other hydrophilic materials are also available for this purpose. The insertion of laminaria 4 to 24 hours before the abortion helps to make dilation of the cervix easier.*

Although many abortions during the first trimester can be done without the use of preoperative laminaria, they are particularly beneficial for second-trimester abortions, which require more dilation of the cervix.

Insertion of laminaria is a 5-minute procedure. The vagina is first cleansed with an antiseptic solution, and a sterile speculum is inserted, just as for a pelvic exam. Next, the cervix is gently grasped with an instrument to stabilize it. At this point, the patient may feel a pinch or cramp. The laminaria are then inserted into the cervical opening. Their presence may cause some cramping as the uterus contracts in response to the foreign object. Antiseptic-soaked gauze sponges are then gently inserted into the vagina (much like a tampon) to help keep the laminaria in place. The speculum is removed and the procedure is over. Discomfort during this insertion is typically limited to mild menstrual-like cramps.

Following laminaria insertion, the patient may experience some modest vaginal bleeding or leakage of antiseptic solution, which necessitates the use of a sanitary napkin. The patient should not have sex or place anything inside the vagina following the insertion of laminaria, including tampons and douche nozzles. It is common to experience some cramping overnight as the cervix dilates; medication used for menstrual cramps, such as ibuprofen, can be helpful. Occasionally, the laminaria may be expelled from the body. If this happens, they should not be reinserted. In most cases, the abortion can be performed as scheduled.

### Procedure

The abortion itself is characteristically performed in an outpatient surgical setting. It can be performed with or without intravenous sedation, although sedation makes the procedure much less unpleasant. At the start of the procedure, a paracervical block with 1% lidocaine is often injected directly into the cervix (4 mL at the 3:00 and 9:00 positions) after the painless removal of the laminaria. Some patients feel a brief, sharp pain during the injection of the medication. From this point, most women experience very little discomfort, although some may have a vague cramping sensation in the lower abdomen. The patient may also hear the whirring sound of the vacuum. The entire abortion, from draping the abdomen to completion of the procedure, usually takes an average of 15 minutes.

After the abortion, the patient remains under medical observation for several hours. Most abortion facilities require that the patient be accompanied by someone when going home, because the medication effects may persist. Patients are occasionally given one or two types of medication to be taken for the next several days. One is methergine 0.2 mg, taken every 4 to 6 hours, to help make the uterus contract (cramp) and thereby reduce blood loss.

*CONTROVERSY: Some practitioners also prescribe several days of antibiotics (typically doxycycline 100 mg twice daily for 5 days) to reduce the risk of infection, although usually this threat is very small. Rh-negative women also receive an intramuscular injection of Rh immune globulin (RhoGAM).*

### Follow-Up

Most women will have some vaginal bleeding for 1 to 2 weeks after the procedure. The bleeding may be associated with some cramping. If the bleeding is heavier than a menstrual period, or if the patient experiences very painful cramping, the practitioner should be notified. Most women will get their first menstrual period 4 to 6 weeks after the abortion, but this timing varies widely. Patients should be instructed to call the health care provider if they develop a fever.

Timing of the postabortion checkup varies; it is often recommended at 2 weeks. The practitioner will check to be sure that the uterus is a normal size and may also prescribe contraceptives, such as the pill or a diaphragm. Until the postoperative exam, sex should be avoided and nothing should be placed in the vagina, including tampons and douches. It is important to remember that a woman can ovulate at any time after an abortion. When intercourse is resumed, some type of contraception should be used if pregnancy is to be avoided.

## Medical Methods of Abortion

There are two basic medical types of abortion: injection of drugs directly into the pregnant uterus and the use of vaginal suppositories. Both use specific types of prostaglandins to cause the uterus to contract. These methods are usually used only for second-trimester abortions and actually cause "labor" in that the uterus contracts and, after a period of time, expels the pregnancy. Before injecting a medication into the uterus, prepare the skin with an antiseptic. A small amount of anesthetic agent is often injected into the abdominal wall. Then, usually with the help of ultrasound guidance, fluid is removed from the uterus by a needle placed through the abdominal wall, and an equal volume of drug is injected. Medications used for this purpose have included hypertonic saline and prostaglandins. There may be a delay of as long as 12 hours between the injection and the beginning of contractions. After the contractions begin, it can take a number of hours to expel the pregnancy. To reduce her discomfort, the patient is typically medicated during this time. Sometimes laminaria are placed in advance to prepare the cervix. Medical induction of abortion sometimes needs to be supplemented with the D&E procedure described earlier if the entire pregnancy is not expelled.

An alternative medical method for causing labor involves the insertion of vaginal suppositories of prostaglandin E. These suppositories, placed every 4 to 6 hours, ultimately result in contractions that expel the pregnancy. This medication, unfortunately, has a variety of side effects, including rapid pulse, low blood pressure, high fever, diarrhea, and nausea. Although liberal use is made of a variety of medications to counteract these side effects, the experience still tends to be uncomfortable. This method is usually reserved for pregnancies in the later second trimester, which are large enough to make a D&E difficult.

## Safety of Abortion

In reviewing the safety of abortion, it may be helpful to remember that the death rate from vaginal birth at term is 10 out of 100,000 women and that the death rate from cesarean section at term for a woman in labor is roughly 40 to 50 out of 100,000. **PEARL: The risk of death from abortion in the first 12 weeks of pregnancy is approximately 1 in 100,000 to 1 in 400,000. From this perspective, abortion is 10 to 40 times safer than simply having a baby.** The risk of death from abortion rises with increasing delay to roughly 18 deaths per 100,000 procedures toward the end of the second trimester. This method is still safer than cesarean section at term—a procedure widely accepted as safe. Also, there is no evidence of a postabortion increase in psychiatric disturbances such as depression.

Although by any standard abortion is a "safe" operation, a number of complications are worth reviewing. First, serious infection can result, requiring hospitalization and treatment with intravenous antibiotics. Such an infection potentially can damage the fallopian tubes, leading to infertility. Second, the uterus can be incompletely emptied, which sometimes results in continued, significant bleeding. This problem is resolved with a second procedure. Conversely, scarring can occur, leading to amenorrhea and secondary infertility (known as Asherman's syndrome). Once in a while, enough blood is lost during the procedure or afterward to require a blood transfusion.

An uncommon but major complication of abortion is damage to one of the abdominal organs. During the procedure, the wall of the uterus may become perforated. Although this perforation often heals without medical intervention, very serious damage can be done if a vital organ or blood vessel is cut or nicked. If the bladder or bowel is injured, a major operation under general anesthesia may be required. Rarely, the major artery supplying the uterus may be ruptured during an abortion, causing a life-threatening hemorrhage that sometimes can be stemmed only by hysterectomy, or removal of the entire uterus. Other uncommon complications of abortion include blood clots and problems with the anesthetic agents.

## Cost of Abortion

The entire cost of a first-trimester abortion at an abortion clinic is only a few hundred dollars. The cost of an early second-trimester abortion is somewhat more. A mid or late second-trimester abortion can run well over $1000. An abortion in a hospital by a private doctor is often two to three times more expensive than a similar procedure performed at an abortion clinic. Although the care may be somewhat less personalized at the clinic, significant economies of scale are chiefly responsible for its lower charge. Also, the fee at the abortion clinic usually does not include the postabortion checkup. Despite the lower cost, access to abortion for poor women has been sharply limited owing to federal restrictions on funding for these procedures through Medicaid.

Many obstetrician-gynecologists do not perform abortions but refer patients to abortion clinics. Although the quality of care can vary at these facilities, the doctors at these clinics are usually very experienced. The complication rate is definitely reduced when the practitioner has more experience with this seemingly straightforward procedure.

## CONTRACEPTIVE SAFETY AND EFFECTIVENESS

If a couple in good health were to begin regular intercourse at about age 21 and did not use contraceptives, they could expect to give birth to an average of 10 children over their lifetimes. This fact has caused most cultures from the beginning of time to develop various customs, taboos, and birth control methods to limit population growth. Tables 3–2 and 3–3 summarize the questions of safety and effectiveness, which are critical considerations for couples making choices about contraceptives.

## Table 3–2. RISKS OF EVERYDAY LIVING, CONCEPTION, AND CONTRACEPTION

| Activity | Chance of Death in 1 Year |
| --- | --- |
| **EVERYDAY ACTIVITY** | |
| Motorcycling | 1 in 1000 |
| Automobile driving | 1 in 6000 |
| Power boating | 1 in 6000 |
| Rock climbing | 1 in 7500 |
| Playing football | 1 in 25,000 |
| Canoeing | 1 in 100,000 |
| Using tampons (toxic shock) | 1 in 350,000 |
| Having sexual intercourse (PID) | 1 in 50,000 |
| **RESOLVING PREGNANCY** | |
| Vaginal birth | 1 in 10,000 |
| Legal abortion before 9 weeks | 1 in 262,000 |
| Legal abortion within 9–12 weeks | 1 in 100,000 |
| Legal abortion within 13–15 weeks | 1 in 34,400 |
| Legal abortion after 15 weeks | 1 in 10,000 |
| **PREVENTING PREGNANCY** | |
| Oral contraception, nonsmoker, <35 years old | 1 in 200,000 |
| Oral contraception, smoker, <35 years old | 1 in 5,300 |
| IUD | 1 in 10,000,000 (per year) |
| Hysterectomy | 1 in 1,600 |
| Laparoscopic tubal ligation | 1 in 38,500 |
| Vasectomy | 1 in 1,000,000 |

IUD = intrauterine device; PID = pelvic inflammatory disease.
**Source:** Adapted from Trussell, J and Kowal, D: The essentials of contraception. In Hatcher, RA, et al: Contraceptive Technology, ed 17. New York, Ardent Publishers, 1998, p 230.

### Table 3–3. EFFECTIVENESS OF VARIOUS CONTRACEPTIVE METHODS*

| Method | Best Rate (%) | Typical Rate (%) |
|---|---|---|
| Total abstinence | 100.0 | 100.0 |
| Norplant | 99.9 | 99.9 |
| Vasectomy | 99.8 | 99.8 |
| Tubal ligation | 99.6 | 99.6 |
| Injectable progestin | 99.5 | 98.0 |
| Combined birth control pill | 99.5 | 98.0 |
| Progestin-only pill | 99.0 | 97.5 |
| IUD | 98.5 | 95.0 |
| Condom | 98.0 | 90.0 |
| Cervical cap | 98.0 | 87.0 |
| Sponge (with spermicide) | 91.0 | 80–90 |
| Diaphragm (with spermicide) | 98.0 | 81.0 |
| Foams, creams, jellies, and vaginal suppositories | 95–97 | 82.0 |
| Coitus interruptus | 84.0 | 77.0 |
| Periodic abstinence | 98.0 | 76.0 |
| Douche | — | 60.0 |
| No contraceptive use | 10.0 | 10.0 |

*The chances of not getting pregnant during 1 year of regular intercourse. The higher the number, the more effective the contraceptive method.

**Source:** Adapted from Russell T and Host: Contraceptive efficacy. In Hatcher, RA et al: Contraceptive Technology, ed 17. New York, Ardent Publishers, 1998, p 800.

# 4

# Vulvar and Vaginal Complaints

After concerns about bleeding, the symptoms most often raised during gynecology visits are complaints about vulvar and vaginal symptoms. Although they often occur together, vaginal discharge and vaginal irritation are actually two separate symptoms. Identifying the chief complaint helps to narrow the list of differential diagnoses.

## VULVAR IRRITATION

Vulvar itching or irritation can, of course, result from vaginal infections with bacteria, but many patients complain of these symptoms without having an abnormal discharge. **PEARL: In these cases, the differential diagnoses are chiefly (1) fungal infections, (2) local skin disease, (3) contact dermatitis, or (4) unknown.**

### Fungal Infections

There are typically two different groups of pathogens: *Candida* species and tinea. The *Candida* infections are commonly known as "yeast." *Candida* infections can cause vulvar irritation with a concomitant increase in vaginal secretions. Tinea, which is much more common in men, is known by the slang "jock itch."

With *Candida* infections, the skin typically shows pustules on an erythematous base, although sometimes only erythema is present. Scratching can produce secondary changes such as cracking. **PEARL: Tinea cruris, which is less common, is characterized by concentric pustules with a more-or-less normal central region.** Neither disease is commonly spread through sexual contact, but treatment of sexual partners may be considered for patients with frequent recurrences. In general, tinea can be treated with the same antifungal agents as *Candida* infections (Table 4–1), although a twice-a-day topical regimen for several weeks is usually necessary to prevent recurrences.

### Table 4–1. TREATMENT OF *CANDIDA* VULVOVAGINITIS

| Brand | Generic | Available Without Prescription? | Directions |
|---|---|---|---|
| Diflucan | Fluconazole | No | 150-mg tablet orally, once |
| Terazol | Terconazole | No | 0.4% vaginal cream—one applicator qhs ×7 <br> 0.8% vaginal cream—one applicator qhs ×3 |
| Femstat | Butoconazole | Yes | Vaginal cream—one applicator qhs ×3 |
| Monistat | Miconzole | Yes | Vaginal cream—one applicator qhs ×7 |
| Vagistat | Tioconazole | Yes | Vaginal cream—one prefilled applicator once |

For those with considerable itching, a mild steroid cream (such as hydrocortisone 2.5%) can be applied concomitantly for 7 days to help speed relief.

## Local Skin Diseases

Occasionally, local skin diseases can present with vulvar itching or burning (Table 4–2). Diagnosis of these conditions is typically made after performing a 3-mm punch biopsy after an injection of local anesthetic. Suturing the site is rarely necessary, and hemostasis usually can be achieved by applying silver nitrate to the wound. Atrophic vaginitis is seen only in postmenopausal women, usually only after years of estrogen deficiency. It ordinarily responds to estrogen within a month or so.

Lichen simplex chronicus results from inflammatory changes in the skin caused by repetitive scratching. It typically follows some inciting event such as a vulvocandidiasis. Lichen sclerosis can occur in men and on other parts of the body, although for reasons unknown, it most commonly presents on the vulva. Its etiology is elusive. Vulvar psoriasis is frequently accompanied by lesions elsewhere on the body. Finally, vulvar intraepithelial neoplasia has been linked to human papillomavirus infections; the relationship between either of these conditions and squamous cell cancer of the vulva remains unclear.

**PEARL: Diabetes can cause a vulvar neuropathy that presents as vulvar burning.** This conditon is relatively rare and is typically seen in insulin-dependent diabetics, although it can occur in women with undiagnosed carbohydrate intolerance. Vigorous blood glucose control may offer some benefit.

## Other Causes of Vulvar Irritation

The most difficult patients to treat are those with idiopathic vulvar irritation, also known as vestibulitis or vulvodynia. Some of these patients are suspected of having a sort of contact dermatitis reaction to some substance in the environment, such as shampoo, soap,

**Table 4–2. LOCAL SKIN DISEASES
AFFECTING THE VULVA**

| Disease | Appearance | Treatment |
|---|---|---|
| Atrophic vaginitis | Thin, pale skin | Estrogen via any route (oral, trans-dermal, vaginal) |
| Lichen simplex chronicus | Thickened, erythematous skin | Highly potent steroid cream (Fluocinonide daily for 3 weeks, then decrease) |
| Lichen sclerosis | White, thin skin with occasionally thickened borders and cracking | Super potent steroid cream (clobetasol proprionate once daily for 4–6 weeks, then decrease) |
| Psoriasis | Thick red, scaly patches with erythema | Highly potent steroid cream (Fluocinonide daily for 3 weeks, then decrease) |
| Condyloma | Flat to papulary flesh-colored lesions | Physical destruction of lesion |
| Vulvar intra-epithelial neoplasia | Typically white epithelium with cracking | Physical destruction of lesion |

detergent, fibers in clothes, or feminine hygiene products—virtually anything that comes in contact with the vulva.

**CONTROVERSY: Unfortunately, there is no way to prove that contact dermatitis is the cause of idiopathic vulvar irritation, and the substance responsible is rarely identified.**

Even if the offending item is identified and removed from the environment, the irritation can take months to resolve. Occasionally, symptomatic relief can be obtained from steroid creams, but these medications should be used only for 2 weeks at a time because prolonged use can cause skin atrophy. Topical steroids can control symptoms of vulvar conditions but do not cure the underlying disease. Overuse can thin the skin, predispose the patient to fungal and bacteria infections, and result in "steroid rebound dermatitis"—a condition that can rival the original disease in discomfort. Lidocaine 5% ointment applied as often as necessary may also be helpful. Most patients, however, simply have to wait several months for the burning sensation to go away.

## VAGINAL DISCHARGE

When a patient's chief complaint is vaginal discharge, ask her about the quantity, color, and presence or absence of odor (Table 4–3). The number of her sexual partners in the previous 12 months is also particularly relevant. Women with three or more partners probably should be checked routinely for gonorrhea and chlamydia.

Vaginal smears are helpful in diagnosing yeast infections, bacterial vaginosis, and trichomoniasis. Any discharge is swabbed with a cotton applicator and then smeared onto a slide, to which one drop of normal saline is applied, followed by one drop of dilute potassium hydroxide next to but separate from the normal saline. Two coverslips are applied, and the slide is then examined under the microscope at low power. Yeast appears as thin branching sticks that occasionally have spores visible as round ball-like structures protruding from the stick. Bacterial vaginosis gives off a pungent, fishy odor when potassium hydroxide is applied and can be further recognized by the presence of clue cells—squamous epithelium covered with tiny specks that are presumably the bacteria clinging to the cell. Bacterial vaginosis results from a shift in vaginal flora toward anaerobic species such as *Gardnerella*, *Mobiluncus*, and *Mycoplasma*. Its cause is not well understood. Finally, trichomonas can occasionally be recognized by observing small, mobile, spherelike structures. The key with trichomonas is to look at the slide quickly because trichomonads rapidly become immobile at

### Table 4–3. COMMON CAUSES OF VAGINAL DISCHARGE

|  | **Candidiasis** | **Bacterial Vaginosis** | **Tricho-moniasis** |
|---|---|---|---|
| Color | White, curdy | Yellow-green | Gray |
| Odor | None | Mild ("fishy" on KOH prep) | Mild |
| Pruritis, burning | Prominent | Minimal | Prominent |
| Vulvar erythema | Prominent | Variable | Minimal |
| Wet mount | Budding hyphae | Clue cells | Motile tricho-monads |
| Treatment | Anti-fungal agents (see Table 4–1) | Metronidazole 500 mg bid × 7 days *OR* 2 g orally as single dose (less effective)* | Metro-nidazole 500 mg bid × 7 days *OR* 2 g orally as single dose (less effective) |

*Alternatives: metronidazole gel 0.75%, one applicator intravaginally bid for 5 days; clindamycin 300 mg bid for 7 days; or clindamycin cream 2%, one applicator qhs for 7 nights.

room temperature, and they are difficult to identify unless they are darting about on the slide. Another clue suggesting trichomonas is the appearance of the "strawberry cervix," a cervix covered with small, discrete red patches.

As a rule, the partners of women with candidiasis and bacterial vaginosis are not treated unless the infections recur within a short period. The partners of those with trichomoniasis should be treated.

Some women complain of an increased discharge in the absence of demonstrable disease. **PEARL: This physiologic increase in vaginal discharge is suggested when the patient has little or no itching or odor, and when the discharge is white or clear.**

One common scenario for this complaint involves a patient who has stopped taking oral contraceptive pills and subsequently experiences an increase in discharge during midcycle with ovulation.

## PAIN ON INTERCOURSE (DYSPAREUNIA)

Pain on intercourse is another common complaint that rarely is the result of an underlying disease process. **PEARL: Distinguish between pain at the vaginal opening, which is usually the result of a local irritation such as that caused by spermicides, and deep dyspareunia.** The usual reason for deep dyspareunia is that the patient is not fully aroused before penile insertion. The first sign of female sexual arousal is profuse vaginal lubrication. The next sign, which occurs a few minutes before orgasm, is expansion of the inner third of the vagina. If the penis is inserted too early in the cycle of female sexual arousal (as it often is), discomfort can be experienced because the vaginal walls are forcefully separated. Treatment consists of simply prolonging foreplay, chiefly clitoral massage. This cause of dyspareunia may be virtually excluded if the pain occurs during sexual intercourse that results in orgasm.

Other causes of dyspareunia include pelvic masses and endometriosis. A pelvic mass causing painful intercourse should be obvious on exam. If endometriosis is the cause, it typically causes localized tenderness on exam similar to what is experienced during intercourse. Even so, endometriosis should not be diagnosed as a cause without laparoscopic confirmation. Many cases of dyspareunia simply do not have an obvious explanation, but the painful episodes resolve with time. In the meantime, patients should be encouraged to try different coital positions.

## BARTHOLIN DUCT ABSCESS

Bartholin's glands are small glands at the opening of the vagina. Their purpose remains a puzzle. Yet these innocuous structures can become a health issue when their openings become plugged and they become secondarily infected. Women with Bartholin gland abscess typically present with an exquisitely tender, fluctuant, swollen mass just lateral to the labia, close to the posterior fourchette. Treatment involves incision and drainage. Because the problem often recurs, the specific procedure depends on the history and becomes more involved as the recurrences go up.

## Incision and Drainage

Typically the easiest procedure, incision and drainage can be performed directly in the clinic and is the first choice for first-time occurrences. Inject a small wheal of local anesthetic into the skin over the abscess and make a 5-mm incision. Allow the pus to drain out. Typically, a wound culture is obtained, although the results are rarely useful because this procedure usually is the only treatment necessary. Then insert a Word catheter through the incision, and inflate the balloon with 2 to 3 mL of normal saline or water. The Word catheter is allowed to remain in place for 6 weeks, but often it falls out sooner on its own. Patients may bathe, but intercourse is problematic because it is likely to dislodge the catheter prematurely.

## Marsupialization

For those with several recurrences, the gland is opened up with an incision that is 2 to 3 cm long. This is typically accomplished with intravenous sedation and local anesthesia. Loculations are broken up bluntly with a hemostat. The gland edges are then sutured to the skin edge in a circumferential manner using a small absorbable suture such as 3–0 chromic. Typically iodoform gauze is used to pack the wound to help keep it open for several days. The gauze is removed 2 or 3 days later, and the patient is allowed to go about normal activities (including bathing). The wound usually closes after several weeks.

## Excision of the Gland

This procedure is typically reserved for those in whom marsupialization fails. Bleeding can be an issue and may require suturing or electrocautery. After the gland is dissected out, the wound typically has to be closed in several layers.

## RETAINED TAMPON

Although it is not often discussed in gynecology texts, a retained tampon is a real-world complaint. **PEARL: Of women who present thinking that they have a retained tampon, at least half do not have anything inside the vagina.** More commonly, women will present with a malodorous discharge. To the novice, a tampon that has been left in place for several days can at first appear to be some sort of tumor. After removal, women usually do not need to do anything more than perhaps douche once with an over-the-counter iodine douche. Contrary to expectations, toxic shock syndrome remains an uncommon occurrence.

## TOXIC SHOCK SYNDROME

Toxic shock syndrome was originally linked to a specific type of tampon. **PEARL: It has since been realized that toxic shock syndrome can result from a variety of clinical situations including diaphragm use, simple skin lesions, and surgical incisions that become infected with specific strains of *Staphylococcus aureus*.**

These strains produce a specific toxin that results in high fever, rash, hypotension, vomiting, and watery diarrhea. Treatment consists of supportive care (generally in an intensive care unit [ICU]), high-dose steroids, and a beta-lactamase–resistant antibiotic with activity against *S. aureus*.

# 5

CHAPTER

# Miscellaneous Gynecologic Problems

A variety of gynecologic problems unrelated to bleeding or vaginal infections arise in the office. Some problems, such as dysmenorrhea or galactorrhea, can be classified as symptoms, whereas others, such as enlarged ovaries, are discovered during the course of a physical exam and are more properly known as "signs."

## PREMENSTRUAL SYNDROME

Lay people use the term premenstrual syndrome (PMS) so indiscriminately that it can mean virtually any symptom, whether it is experienced cyclically or not.

**PEARL: When patients inquire about PMS, you should obtain a more detailed history before making any recommendations.**

The medical definition of PMS is one or more symptoms occurring at a fixed time in every menstrual cycle, typically within a week before menses and lasting for only a few days. More than 100 symptoms have been ascribed to PMS; they include moodiness, emotional lability, depression, nausea, pelvic congestion or pain, diarrhea, bloating, swelling, fatigue, insomnia, headaches, and food cravings. Several dozen specific substances measurable in the peripheral blood have been studied, and no correlation has been found between the blood level of any chemical or hormone and the symptoms. Yet with so many people presenting with similar complaints, the phenomenon of premenstrual distress in some women is probably a biologically real event. The problem is that we simply do not understand the process yet and therefore have no reliable treatment method.

The first approach to PMS is to clarify the patient's symptoms, particularly their timing. Ideally, patients should keep a symptom log through three cycles, although few comply with this advice. Treatment then depends on the symptom. For premenstrual swelling, a diuretic can be used for up to 7 days a month. Bloating or abdominal distension has no specific treatment. It may result when progesterone produced after ovulation inhibits the smooth muscle motility of the small intestine. Pain and diarrhea may be treated with nonsteroidal anti-inflammatory drugs.

Depression and moodiness need intense scrutiny. **PEARL: Many patients who complain of premenstrual depression are actually depressed and simply experiencing the waxing and waning of the illness. These patients usually respond well to antidepressants; indeed, some have recommended the routine use of antidepressants to treat premenstrual moodiness or despair.** In general, it is most useful to view these patients as depressed (an illness relatively well understood) rather than to assign them a diagnosis with no effective treatment. Many patients, however, prefer to think of their condition as PMS rather than as depression. Perhaps this is because depression is often viewed as a classic psychiatric diagnosis with its attendant stigma, whereas PMS may be a more socially acceptable condition. As a rule, only the most discomfited patients accept a diagnosis of depression and follow up with a psychiatrist.

General advice that can be given to women with PMS is to avoid caffeine during the week before the menses and to be sure to get appropriate amounts of sleep. This involves going to bed at the same time each night and waking up at the same time each morning.

## DECREASED LIBIDO

A major reason, if the not the biggest single cause, for decreased libido in female patients is disaffection with their mate's behavior. The offending actions can range from physical abuse to inattention. Although it may seem strange, many women seem surprised to hear that their sexual urges may be suppressed because they are angry at their sexual partner. This symptom of a troubled relationship is very difficult to treat, but providing this simple insight may sometimes prove helpful. **PEARL: A depressed sex drive by itself is almost never the sole manifestation of other diseases.** Changing or stopping oral contraceptives rarely affects libido. In evaluating decreased libido, it is important to take a sexual history with emphasis on coital frequency, past and present. The average coital frequency for a married couple is 7.5 times per month. Of course, this number varies considerably from couple to couple, and obtaining information about a change in frequency may be helpful.

**PEARL: Another common reason for decreased libido is depression.** A careful history will show that a depressed sex drive is almost never the only symptom of depression. If the history suggests that depression is a likely cause, antidepressant medication or psychiatric referral is usually the most appropriate treatment approach. Virtually any disease process can depress the sex drive, either directly or through psychological distress. In general, other symptoms or physical findings will point to a specific cause.

*CONTROVERSY: The use of topical or oral testosterone to improve libido remains controversial because of the lack of data supporting efficacy. Also, all methods and doses of testosterone supplementation commonly prescribed for women are linked to a dose-related risk of side effects including hirsutism, acne, clitoromegaly, and deepening of the voice.*

## GALACTORRHEA

A milky-white breast discharge, whether from one or both breasts, is known as galactorrhea and should be distinguished from other nipple secretions, which may be green or bloody, for instance. **PEARL: Galactorrhea generally is idiopathic, medication induced, or a result of hyperprolactinemia.** Idiopathic galactorrhea is obviously a diagnosis of exclusion. Medications that can cause galactorrhea include oral contraceptive pills, amphetamines, and tricyclic antidepressants.

The initial evaluation of a patient with galactorrhea should include levels of thyroid-stimulating hormone (TSH) and prolactin (Fig. 5–1). Elevated levels of TSH may reflect increased production of thyroid-releasing hormone (TRH) within the hypothalamus. TRH is thought to double as a prolactin-releasing factor, and certain hypothyroid states are associated with galactorrhea. In these cases, correcting the thyroid malfunction will cure the galactorrhea. Alternatively, an elevation in prolactin can suggest a benign pituitary tumor. If the initial screening prolactin level is only borderline high, it should be repeated in the fasting state. If the second one is high or the first was significantly elevated, magnetic resonance imaging (MRI) or a computed tomography (CT) scan of the pituitary should be obtained to

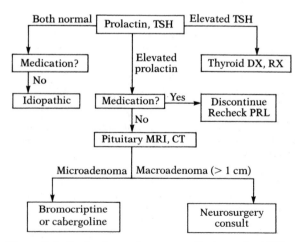

**Figure 5–1.** Evaluation and treatment of galactorrhea. PRL = prolactin; TSH = thyroid-stimulating hormone.

rule out a large pituitary tumor. Large tumors (less than 1 cm in diameter) can injure the optic nerve and occasionally require neurosurgical reduction as well as medication.

One of the medications used to treat hyperprolactinemia is bromocriptine (Parlodel). As a dopamine agonist, this drug is very effective in lowering prolactin levels and occasionally even in shrinking pituitary adenomas. Unfortunately, because of its significant side effects, such as dizziness on standing and nausea, the initial dose must be small. One regimen is to cut 2.5-mg pills in half and take 1.25 mg each night for 2 weeks, followed first by 2.5 mg each night for 2 weeks, and then by 2.5 mg twice daily. The prolactin level is rechecked after 4 weeks of a steady dose of Parlodel, and the dosage can be adjusted as necessary. Patients should be reminded not to check their nipples for discharge because this practice tends to prolong the galactorrhea.

*CONTROVERSY: For those few patients who cannot tolerate this gradual regimen, the same result can be achieved by simply placing the pills into the vagina instead of taking them orally. For some, this seems to eliminate most of the side effects while reducing prolactin levels.*

It is wise to recheck the prolactin levels periodically, at least yearly. The dose for long-term maintenance should be reduced to the lowest amount of Parlodel that keeps the prolactin level normal. Some patients require only one quarter of a tablet daily.

*CONTROVERSY: Once the prolactin has returned to normal on the Parlodel, the duration of treatment remains debated. Some specialists advocate long-term suppression, because these tumors can regrow after cessation of treatment.*

Elevated prolactin levels are also associated with menstrual disruptions and anovulation. Infertility patients with hyperprolactinemia occasionally resume ovulating simply after treatment with Parlodel.

A new alternative to Parlodel is cabergoline (Dostinex). Supplied in scored 0.5-mg tablets, the initial dose is 0.25 mg twice a week with increases in increments of 0.25 mg, up to 1 mg twice a week. A prolactin level should be checked after 4 weeks at each new dosage. Side effects include orthostatic hypotension, headache, nausea, and vomiting. The manufacturer suggests that the drug should be discontinued 6 months after a normal prolactin level has been obtained, with subsequent monitoring of the level to be sure it remains normal.

## HIRSUTISM

**PEARL: Most complaints about excessive hair growth are the result of a familial or constitutional tendency toward hirsutism.** Unfortunately, aside from electrolysis, waxing, and chemical depilatories, little in the way of a permanent curative treatment exists. Laser ablation of hair follicles may be beneficial, but the treatment is relatively new and initial reports are mixed.

On occasion, a patient will have an underlying endocrine disorder that is treatable. Because the complaint of hirsutism is highly subjective, the history should focus on recent increases in hair growth and the hair distribution of family members, particularly parents. Ultimately, however, the decision to do a workup is a judgment call. Other clues to excessive androgen production include acne and oily skin. Advanced symptoms of masculinization include voice deepening and clitoral enlargement.

**PEARL: Androgens are produced by both the ovary and the adrenal gland.** Each of these organs directly produces about 25% of circulating testosterone, whereas peripheral tissue conversion of androstenedione (90% secreted by the adrenal) accounts for the remainder. The adrenal gland also produces an additional androgen, dehydroepiandrosterone sulfate (DHEAS).

Several derangements can result in symptoms of androgen excess. Testosterone or DHEAS can be produced in excess because of either an endocrine disorder or a benign or malignant neoplasm. Alternatively, the amount of free androgen in the circulation can be increased through a problem with sex hormone–binding globulin. Finally, the end-organ tissues can have increased sensitivity to androgens.

The screening tests for hirsutism are a testosterone level (total, free, and bound) and a DHEAS level (Fig. 5–2). Total testosterone levels >200 ng/dL suggest an ovarian tumor and should be followed up by a CT scan and possibly an exploratory laparotomy. DHEAS levels greater than 700 μg/dL require an adrenal suppression test with 4 days of dexamethasone and repeat DHEAS level tests. Failure to lower the DHEAS level in this manner suggests an adrenal tumor.

**PEARL: Mildly elevated levels of both total testosterone and DHEAS can be suppressed with oral contraceptive pills, although the effect on DHEAS is not well understood.** In addition to directly suppressing production of these hormones, the estrogen component of the pill causes an increase in the sex hormone–binding globulin, which, in turn, reduces the availability of testosterone.

An additional approach to treatment is to reduce end-organ sensitivity by a trial of spironolactone. It binds to androgen receptor sites and inhibits the enzyme (5-

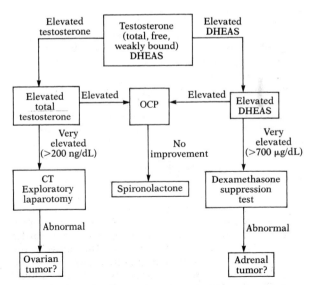

**Figure 5–2.** Evaluation and treatment of hirsutism. OCP = oral contraceptive pill.

alpha reductase) that converts testosterone to the more potent dihydrotestosterone in the target tissue. A mild diuretic, spironolactone can be given in doses of 25 mg up to four times a day for an extended period. Patients should be tapered off the medication over several weeks when they wish to stop it.

Rarely, hirsutism can be the presenting symptom of Cushing's syndrome, which is caused by the overproduction of cortisol. This diagnosis can be excluded by a single 1-mg dose of dexamethasone at bedtime, followed by a plasma cortisol measurement the next morning. Values of less than 6 $\mu$g/dL effectively rule out Cushing's syndrome.

## PELVIC PAIN

In general, the diagnostic possibilities for patients presenting with pelvic pain can be greatly narrowed simply by taking a history. Location, duration, severity, association with vaginal bleeding, exacerbating factors, and other symptoms—particularly fever and gastrointestinal complaints—will all help to focus the investigation. For classification purposes, pelvic pain is considered chronic when it has lasted for 6 months or more.

Given the frequency of pregnancy-related problems, a pregnancy test is often a wise choice in women of reproductive age. The presence or absence of fever helps in determining the presence of an infectious etiology. Pelvic examination can help determine the likelihood of uterine or ovarian involvement. Laparoscopy to establish the presence of adhesions or endometriosis should generally be reserved for use later in the investigation. Occasionally, especially for those with chronic pelvic pain, no specific etiology is found and medical management will have to suffice.

# 2
**PART**

*Specialty Clinics*

# 6
## CHAPTER

# *Urogynecology Clinic*

## PROLAPSE

### Definitions

**PEARL: Over time, the connective tissue supports of the pelvic organs can lose their elasticity, resulting in a herniation of the uterus, bladder, or rectum into the vagina and even through the vaginal opening.** Bladder prolapse through the anterior wall of the vagina is known as a cystocele; urethrocele is a term for urethral descent. Rectal herniation through the posterior wall of the vagina is similarly known as a rectocele. There is no specialized term for uterine prolapse except in the specific circumstance in which the entire organ has fallen through the vaginal opening—a condition known as procidentia. An enterocele occurs behind the cervix or near the top of the vagina and refers to a herniation of the small intestine into the vagina. One of the difficulties in characterizing prolapse is the lack of a uniform definition.

**PEARL: Defining the degree of descent in prolapse is made problematic by the variations in normal anatomy and the lack of a strong correlation from patient to patient between amount of herniation and symptoms.** One example of a grading system is shown in Table 6–1.

### Table 6–1. GRADING SYSTEM
### FOR ORGAN PROLAPSE

| Stage | Level of Descent of the Prolapsed Organ |
|-------|------------------------------------------|
| 0 | No descent |
| 1 | Halfway to the hymen |
| 2 | To the hymen |
| 3 | Halfway through the hymen |
| 4 | Completely through the hymen |

## Symptoms

Patient symptoms with prolapse are typically pain or pressure, particularly when standing. Women may also complain of "something protruding" through the vagina with activity. With extreme rectal prolapse, some women actually have to push the back wall of the vagina into position simply to defecate. Bladder prolapse can result in a specific and troubling type of urinary incontinence, which occurs with rises in abdominal pressure such as with coughing, laughing, sneezing, or exercise.

## Surgical Treatment

Various operations have been developed to deal with the different types of prolapse.

### Rectocele

Known as a posterior colporraphy, the procedure to correct a rectocele involves dissecting the vaginal mucosa off the underlying rectovaginal fascia (which is tenuous and often difficult to identify). The excess vaginal tissue is excised, and the underlying fascia is brought together in the midline by placing sutures as far laterally as possible and tying them together. The vaginal mucosa is then reapproximated by sutures.

## *Enterocele*

This hernia is typically encountered during other vaginal surgery. The emphasis in its repair is on identifying the peritoneal sac containing the small intestine, dissecting and excising it, and then closing it in a purse-string fashion. When possible, the uterosacral ligaments are sutured together to help prevent a recurrence.

## *Uterine Prolapse*

The most common operation for uterine prolapse is a vaginal hysterectomy. For patients who are too infirm to tolerate a hysterectomy and who are no longer sexually active, an alternative for the treatment of uterine prolapse is to obliterate the vagina. The most common procedure for this is the LeFort operation, in which the partially denuded anterior and posterior walls of the vagina are sewn together. A small canal is left in the middle of the vagina for the egress of mucus and secretions.

One of the issues in the treatment of uterine prolapse is the possibility that the vaginal vault itself will prolapse in the years to come. Experience suggests that this is more likely in those women suffering from procidentia, the complete extrusion of the uterus through the vaginal introitus. For patients with procidentia, or those with a vault prolapse after a hysterectomy, two surgical approaches can be used:

- **Vaginal approach:** The sacrospinous vault suspension anchors the top of the vagina to the sacrospinous ligament through nonabsorbable sutures.
- **Abdominal approach:** The vault can be suspended either by suturing it to artificial graft material, which is, in turn, sutured to the sacrum, or by freeing up strips of an abdominal fascia and using these to suspend the vagina.

## URINARY INCONTINENCE

**PEARL: Continence is maintained when the pressure of the urethra exceeds the pressure of the bladder.** During micturition, the detrusor muscles of the bladder contract while the urethra relaxes. The bladder contains only smooth muscle; the urethra has a mixture of smooth muscle and striated muscle.

Four types of peripheral nerves influence continence:

- Parasympathetic (S2–S4): Cholinergic stimulation results in bladder contraction.
- Sympathetic (T10–L2) alpha-adrenergic: Activation increases urethral pressure.
- Sympathetic (T10–L2) beta-adrenergic: Activation decreases bladder tone.
- Skeletal (Pudendal nerve, S2–S4): Voluntarily increases urethral pressure.

Our understanding of the neurology of micturation is incomplete, but it is clear that the central nervous system (CNS) also influences continence. A classic example is the urinary retention that can be a presenting symptom of multiple sclerosis.

## Types

Urinary incontinence in women can be classified into several relatively common types:

- **Stress incontinence.** Even though the urethra is functioning normally and the bladder muscles are not contracting, a sudden increase in abdominal pressure (such as with sneezing, laughter, or exercise) can produce urinary incontinence. This type of incontinence typically results from a cystocele. With the bladder dropping out of the true pelvis, the increase in abdominal pressure is transmitted to the top of the bladder but not to its base, so urine is forced out. Paradoxically, the presence of a cystocele does not reliably predict stress incontinence, however. Also, those with extreme bladder descent (through the vaginal opening) may be continent because kinking of the urethra occurs with rises in abdominal pressure.
- **Detrusor instability ("urge" incontinence).** Uncontrolled contractions of the bladder musculature can lead to involuntary expulsion of urine. These bladder spasms can occur randomly but can also be triggered by activity, increases in abdominal pressure, or merely a filling bladder. This type is

also known as "overactive bladder." Symptoms include frequent voidings during the day and getting up to void more than once per night.

- **Low-pressure urethra.** When the urethra is unable to generate normal pressures associated with continence, the symptoms and findings often resemble stress incontinence.

**CONTROVERSY: *There is no universally accepted definition of a low-pressure urethra. A common one is a urethra unable to generate a pressure more than 20 cm of water above bladder resting pressure.***

Low-pressure urethras may result from denervation of the urethra during surgical procedures (including those undertaken to correct incontinence), treatment with radiation to the pelvis, or aging.

- **Overflow incontinence.** The classic symptoms of this condition are uncontrollable dribbling of urine and the inability to generate a strong urine stream. They result from a chronically overfilled bladder. The cause may be obstruction of the urethra (such as by a tumor) or bladder hypotonia, typically from neurologic disease either in the CNS or the peripheral nerves innervating the bladder.

- **Continuous incontinence.** Constant urine loss with the concomitant inability to void significant amounts is suggestive of a urinary tract fistula. The fistulous tract can occur almost anywhere in the urinary system and most commonly exits through the vagina. Fistulas can be a result of malignancies, surgical injuries, or complications of radiation treatment.

## Diagnostic Workup

Because the scientific understanding of incontinence is still incomplete, there is debate about the extent of the workup and the utility of specific studies. Of course, the first place to begin is with a history and physical.

### *History and Voiding Log*

A history directed toward a complaint of urinary incontinence should focus on:

- Frequency (episodes per day/week/month)
- Volume lost
- Precipitating events
- Trend (same, better, worse)
- Number of voids per day
- Number of voids during sleep (nocturia)
- Past medical history including pregnancies and pelvic or vaginal surgery and radiation
- Current medications
- Anal incontinence (flatus or stool)

Another way to obtain historical information is to have the patient keep a voiding diary, or log, for several days. She can keep a prospective record of when she drinks and how much, when she voids, when she leaks, and what else was happening at the time of the incontinent episode.

The idea of the voiding log can be taken further by having the patient measure the voided volumes through the use of a commercially available urine collecting basin (also known as a "hat" for its shape) and even by giving her preweighed pads to use and return in a sealed plastic bag. These can be weighed in their wet state to give a quantitative estimate of urine loss. As a practical matter, however, precise voiding volumes and quantitative estimates of urine loss rarely provide significant additional information in a clinical setting, although they may be useful for research.

### *Physical Examination*

The physical exam is rarely diagnostic by itself, but like the history, it can narrow the possibilities. Findings of particular interest include:

- Abdominal scars
- Abdominal masses
- Presence and degree of herniation into the vagina of bladder, uterus, small bowel, or rectum
- Pelvic masses (paticularly enlargements of uterus or ovaries)
- Anal tone
- Presence of a fistula (occasionally visible or palpable)

### Simple Diagnostic Tests

There are several helpful tests that do not require elaborate equipment and can be performed routinely in the office:

- **Post-void residual.** The volume of urine remaining in the bladder after voiding is measured by straight catheterization of the patient within a few minutes after a void. Volumes less than 50 mL are generally considered normal; those more than 200 mL are thought to represent urinary retention. (There is no consensus on the meaning of volumes between these values.) Those with urinary retention should generally receive a workup focusing on neurologic conditions. Residuals of more than 50 mL may also be seen in women with large cystoceles.

- **Q-tip test.** In this test, a Q-tip covered with 5% lidocaine gel is gently inserted into the urethra to the level of the bladder neck. With the patient in the lithotomy position, the resting angle of the Q-tip relative to the floor is then noted, followed by a measurement of the straining angle. A normal value is an angle change of 30 degrees or less. A greater change indicates urethral hypermobility and suggests stress incontinence.

- **Witnessed incontinence episode.** Women complaining of incontinence can be asked to perform a provocative maneuver such as coughing or bouncing on their heels while they have a full bladder and the urethral meatus is under direct observation. It seems to be a particularly good idea to witness incontinence before performing any surgical corrective procedure.

- **Urinalysis.** This test is used to screen for bacteriuria or hematuria. Those with unexplained hematuria might benefit from an additional urologic workup, including sending urine for cytology.

### Advanced Testing

Some patients with difficult or complex problems of incontinence undergo more sophisticated urodynamic testing. This term does not appear to have a precise meaning but rather refers to one or more of the following tests.

> **CONTROVERSY: The indications for additional testing and the value of these urodynamic tests are particularly controversial. It seems reasonable to conduct further testing on women with previous pelvic surgery (particularly for incontinence), those older than 60, and those with mixed symptoms such as frequent nocturia and incontinence with coughing.**

## Cystometry

Cystometry involves measuring one or more pressures related to voiding as the bladder is being filled with either carbon dioxide gas or a fluid such as saline. Three common pressures are measured either simultaneously or consecutively: bladder pressure, intra-abdominal pressure, and urethral pressure. The sensing devices can employ water manometry, intraluminal computer chips, or other technologies.

Some peculiar terminology is often associated with such testing. Specifically, the term "channel" refers to the number of outputs—not the number of inputs—continously recorded by the measuring device. A typical graphical output would be arrayed as:

Channel 1: Bladder (detrusor) pressure
Channel 2: Intra-abdominal pressure (sensor in either vagina or rectum)
Channel 3: Urethral pressure
Channel 4: True detrusor pressure (bladder pressure minus intra-abdominal pressure)
Channel 5: True urethral pressure (urethral pressure minus intra-abdominal pressure)
Channel 6: True urethral pressure minus true bladder pressure (if a negative number, urine should be lost)

During the cystometrogram, the patient is asked to indicate when she first senses that the bladder is filling ("first sensation"), when she normally would void ("second sensation"), and when she can no longer tolerate further filling ("third sensation"). There are no universally accepted "normals" for these values; most women can hold 500 mL of fluid in their bladder. In evaluating incontinence with cystometry, the patient is often asked to perform provocative procedures, such as coughing or dropping on her heels, to replicate the conditions in which urine is lost. Occasionally, these maneuvers trigger a detrusor contraction that can be measured, thereby distinguishing detrusor instability from genuine stress incontinence. (The term "genuine stress incontinence" denotes an objectively measured drop in urethral pressure below bladder pressure with "stress" such as a cough, as opposed to the symptoms of stress incontinence.)

### Urethral Pressure Measurements

These measurements are obtained by slowly withdrawing the pressure-sensing catheter along the urethra. The difference between the maximum urethral pressure and the resting bladder pressure is known as the maximum urethral closure pressure. Values less than 20 cm of water suggest a diagnosis of "low-pressure urethra." The functional length of the urethra can also be measured in this way.

### Other Tests

Uroflowmetry consists of timing the length and volume of voiding. This process can be done simply with a graduated urine collection basin and a stopwatch or with electronic devices. Generally this test is more useful for men with prostatic hypertrophy, but it is occasionally helpful for women who complain of hesitancy.

Urethrocystoscopy entails observing the mucosal surface of the urethra and bladder and noting the mobility of the urethrovesical junction during provocative maneuvers such as coughing. Lack of mobility may suggest a "frozen" urethra, which is treated somewhat differently than a simple case of urinary stress incontinence.

*CONTROVERSY: The value of uroflowmetry and urethrocystoscopy in the general population is disputed because they rarely add insight.*

## Treatment

The two most common types of incontinence are stress incontinence and detrusor instability. Stress incontinence is usually treated with surgery. The chief objective is to suspend the bladder neck so that it does not drop with increases in abdominal pressure. Dozens of surgical approaches have been described in both the urology and gynecology literature. Vaginal procedures such as the anterior colporraphy have relatively low success rates in terms of the percentage of patients benefiting and the length of benefit.

**CONTROVERSY:** *Needle suspension procedures, in which a long surgical needle is used to suture material from the abdominal fascia (such as above the pubis) to various anchor points beneath the vaginal mucosa, seem to be more effective than a simple anterior colporrhaphy.*

Another group of procedures, known as retropubic urethral suspensions, involves a formal abdominal incision. In the Marshall-Marchetti-Krantz procedure, the anterior wall of the urethra is actually sewn to the back of the symphysis. In the Burch procedure, the tissues lateral to the urethra are sewn to Cooper's ligament (the fascial tissue just above the pubic rami) with either absorbable or nonabsorbable sutures.

**CONTROVERSY:** *The Burch procedure has been described as a laparoscopic technique, but skepticism remains about the duration of its efficacy.*

Detrusor instability (urge incontinence, overactive bladder) usually is treated with medication. Often, the efficacy of these drugs is only moderate and the side effects can be significant. Table 6–2 summarizes the facts about each drug.

Other treatments sometimes used for various types of incontinence include:

- **Bladder training.** This technique can occasionally help those with low bladder capacities and detrusor instability. Patients make a conscious effort to increase their bladder capacity over time by increasing the minimal intervals between voids.
- **Pelvic muscle exercises.** This technique is largely used to help those with stress incontinence. The muscles of the pelvic floor can be strengthened by having the patient perform Kegel exercises or hold

**Table 6–2. MEDICATIONS FOR DETRUSOR INSTABILITY ("OVERACTIVE BLADDER")**

| Generic Name (Brand Name) | Dosage | Mechanism of Action | Side Effects | Contraindications |
|---|---|---|---|---|
| Propantheline bromide 15 mg (Pro-Banthline) | 1 tablet bid to 2 tablets qid | Anticholinergic | Dry mouth, reduced sweating, tachycardia, blurred vision, constipation, urinary retention | Narrow-angle glaucoma, intestinal obstruction, ulcerative colitis, myasthenia gravis |
| Hyoscyamine 0.15 mg (extended release 0.375 mg) (Cystospaz) | 1 or 2 tablets up to qid; extended release, q12h | Anticholinergic | Dry mouth, reduced sweating, tachycardia, blurred vision, constipation, urinary retention | Narrow-angle glaucoma, intestinal obstruction, ulcerative colitis, myasthenia gravis |
| Tolterodine tartrate 1- or 2-mg tablets (Detrol)* | One tablet (2 mg) bid | Anticholinergic (drug of choice among anticholinergics) | Dry mouth, reduced sweating, blurred vision, constipation | Urinary retention, narrow-angle glaucoma, gastric retention |
| Oxybutynin chloride, 5 mg (Ditropan) | 1/2 tablet bid to 1 tablet qid | Antispasmodic, anticholinergic | Dry mouth, reduced sweating, tachycardia, blurred vision, constipation, urinary retention | Narrow-angle glaucoma, intestinal obstruction, ulcerative colitis, myasthenia gravis |

*Continued on following page*

## Table 6–2. MEDICATIONS FOR DETRUSOR INSTABILITY ("OVERACTIVE BLADDER") (*continued*)

| Generic Name (Brand Names) | Dosage | Mechanism of Action | Side Effects | Contraindications |
|---|---|---|---|---|
| Dicyclomine hydrochloride, 10 mg (Bentyl) | 1 tablet bid to 4 tablets qid | Antispasmodic, anticholinergic | Dry mouth, reduced sweating, tachycardia, blurred vision, constipation, urinary retention | Narrow-angle glaucoma, intestinal obstruction, ulcerative colitis, myasthenia gravis |
| Flavoxate hydrochloride 100 mg (Urispas) | 1 or 2 tablets tid–qid | Antispasmodic | Dry mouth, tachycardia, blurred vision | Intestinal obstruction, urinary retention |
| Nifedipine 10 mg (Procardia) | 10 mg bid to 30 mg qid | Calcium channel blocker | Edema, flushing, nausea, headache | Congestive heart failure, severe hypotension or increasing angina after starting drug |
| Imipramine pamoate hydrochloride 75, 100, 125, 150 mg (Tofranil-PM) | 75 mg to 150 mg daily | Adrenergic agonist, anticholinergic | Palpitations, confusion, dry mouth | Concomitant use of MAO inhibitors, arrhythmias, glaucoma |

*Detrol is probably the drug of first choice at this time owing to its relatively improved efficacy and reduced incidence of side effects in comparison with other medications.
MAO = monoamine oxidase.

progressively heavier weighted cones within the vagina.

- **Electrical stimulation.**

*CONTROVERSY: Electrical discharges through intravaginal devices can increase urethral tone by producing a contraction of weakened muscles. This largely experimental procedure is used mainly to treat stress incontinence.*

- **Obstructive devices.** These devices are primarily indicated for those with stress incontinence. A urethral plug can be fitted, which can be worn for several hours. An external string permits removal by deflating the balloon at the end of this short catheter. Another device being developed is a removable, external urethral patch, which also provides a physical barrier to the escape of urine.

# 7
## CHAPTER

# *Sexually Transmitted Disease Clinic*

Although two sexually transmitted diseases that were the bane of the first half of the twentieth century, gonorrhea and syphilis, have started to decline in the United States, other infections such as chlamydia and human immunodeficiency virus (HIV) have arisen to take their place. Those who remark that the emergence of HIV marks "the first time you could have sex and die" are wrong. Before penicillin in the 1930s, syphilis was often fatal. It had been recognized to have something to do with sexual behavior long before bacteria were discovered.

This chapter begins with a table presenting the diagnosis and treatment of 17 sexually transmitted diseases. Five of the diseases—hepatitis B, herpes, HIV infection, pelvic inflammatory disease, and syphilis—are then explained in greater detail.

## AN INVENTORY OF SEXUALLY TRANSMITTED DISEASES

Although the diseases on Table 7–1 are called "sexually transmitted diseases," many of them can be transmitted nonsexually. **PEARL: Scabies and pubic lice, for**

**Table 7-1. SEXUALLY TRANSMITTED DISEASES**

| Disease (Microbe) | Symptoms/Signs | Diagnosis | Treatment | Complications/Comments |
|---|---|---|---|---|
| Bacterial vaginosis (polymicrobial, formerly known as Gardnerella vaginitis). (See also Chapter 4) | Vaginal irritation, discharge, odor Exam: yellow-green discharge with varying degrees of vulvar irritation | Wet mount: clue cells, "fishy" odor on KOH prep pH >4.5 | 1. Metronidazole 500 mg bid × 7 days<br>2. 2 g orally as single dose (less effective)<br>3. Metronidazole gel 0.75% one applicator intravaginally bid for 5 days<br>4. Clindamycin 300 mg bid for 7 days *or* clindamycin cream 2% one applicator qHS for 7 nights | Treat partner for frequent recurrences |
| Chancroid (*Haemophilus ducreyi*) | One or more painful genital ulcers Exam: regional lymphadenopathy | Culture of *H. ducreyi* on special media; negative RPR > 7 days after ulcer onset; HSV culture negative | 1. Azithromycin 1 g once<br>2. Ceftriaxone 250 mg IM once<br>3. Ciprofloxacin 500 mg bid × 3 days<br>4. Erythromycin base 500 mg orally qid × 7 days | Some response usually evident by 3 days; scarring may persist. Considered risk factor for HIV. Coinfection rates with syphilis and herpes significant |

**Table 7-1. SEXUALLY TRANSMITTED DISEASES** (*continued*)

| Disease (Microbe) | Symptoms/Signs | Diagnosis | Treatment | Complications/Comments |
|---|---|---|---|---|
| Chlamydia (*Chlamydia trachomatis*) | Vaginal discharge, dysuria, symptoms of PID<br>Exam: pus in cervix, tender uterus | Culture, immuno-fluorescence assay, DNA probe | Azithromycin 1 g orally once *or* doxycycline 100 mg bid for 7 days | PID, tubal damage |
| Condyloma acuminatum (human papillomavirus). (See also Chapter 8) | Flesh-colored papules, occurring singly or in clusters; sole presenting symptom may be vulvar irritation or itching<br>Exam: Atypical appearance can include erythema or cracking (requires biopsy for diagnosis) | Appearance usually sufficient; skin biopsy when in doubt | *Applied by health professional:*<br>Bi-chloroacetic acid or tri-chloroacetic acid directly to lesions once a week; cryocautery of lesions; excisional biopsy<br>*Applied by patient:*<br>Podofilox 0.5% gel bid × 3 days in weekly cycles up to 4 weeks *or* Imiquimod 5% cream 3 times a week up to 16 weeks | Objective of treating visible external condylomata is elimination of symptoms—no known effect on cervical cancer risk |

| Gonorrhea (*Neisseria gonorrhoeae*) | Vaginal discharge, dysuria, symptoms of PID Exam: pus in cervix, tender uterus | Culture, immunofluorescence assay, DNA probe | Ciprofloxacin 500 mg orally once *or* Ceftriaxone 125 mg IM once (concomitant treatment for chlamydia also advisable) | PID, tubal damage |
|---|---|---|---|---|
| Granuloma inguinale (*Calymmatobacterium granulomatis*) | Painless, beefy red ulcers Exam: Absence of inguinal lymphadenopathy | Biopsy: visualization of Donovan bodies (rare in the United States) | Trimethoprim-sulfamethoxazole double strength *or* doxycycline 100 mg bid until all lesions heal (no less than 3 weeks) | Relapse can occur up to 18 months later |
| Hepatitis B | Jaundice, fever, abdominal pain Exam: hepatomegaly | See text | See text | Liver cancer, chronic illness, potentially fatal |

*Continued on following page*

**Table 7-1. SEXUALLY TRANSMITTED DISEASES (*continued*)**

| Disease (Microbe) | Symptoms/Signs | Diagnosis | Treatment | Complications/ Comments |
|---|---|---|---|---|
| Herpes simplex | Painful blisters on genitals; multiple (usually) grouped vesicles filled with clear fluid that become tender ulcers on erythematous base | Characteristic lesions on exam *Or* viral culture of lesion (sensitivity of culture varies with stage of lesion: 25% before formation of vesicles, 90% with vesicles, and 25% during healing) | See text | Recurrent ulcers; neonatal illness, disability, and death (from vertical transmission at birth—quite rare); serologic testing not helpful for diagnosing genital ulcers (high background rate of exposure) |
| HIV (human immunodeficiency virus) infection | Weight loss, fever, lymphadenopathy, signs of opportunistic infections | HIV antibody as screen. Positive tests require specialty consultation | See text | Potentially fatal |

| | Signs/Symptoms | Diagnosis | Treatment | Complications |
|---|---|---|---|---|
| Lice (*Phthirus pubis*) | Pruritis in groin; visible lice (black motile specks) or nits (white eggs) | Physical exam. Pubic lice can grasp wider hair shafts than head lice; pubic lice can move to head but head lice cannot move to groin | Permethrin 1% cream to affected areas for 10 minutes *or* lindane 1% shampoo for 4 minutes *or* Pyrethrins with piperonyl butoxide for 10 minutes (Medications to be washed off thoroughly after prescribed application) | Thoroughly wash clothing and bedding at high temperature or dry clean; lice on eyelashes require occlusive ophthalmic ointment bid × 10 days |
| Lymphogranuloma inguinale (*Chlamydia trachomatis* strains L1, 2, 3) | Tender, unilateral groin lymphadenopathy. Inflammation in adjacent tissue can result in strictures and fistulas | Serology for chlamydia and exclusion of other causes of lymphadenopathy and ulcers | Doxycycline 100 mg BID for 3 weeks | Fistulas |
| Molluscum contagiosum (*Molluscum contagiosum* virus) | Umbilicated, non-tender papules <5mm with pearly white centers | Biopsy if in doubt | Often resolves without treatment; cryotherapy or caustic chemicals (see Condyloma acuminatum) | — |

*Continued on following page*

## Table 7–1. SEXUALLY TRANSMITTED DISEASES (*continued*)

| Disease (Microbe) | Symptoms/Signs | Diagnosis | Treatment | Complications/Comments |
|---|---|---|---|---|
| Pelvic inflammatory disease (polymicrobial) | Pelvic pain, vaginal discharge, fever Exam: Pus in cervix, tender uterus, tender adnexa, adnexal masses | Elevated white count or sedimentation rate, positive cervical cultures | See text | Tubal damage and infertility, pelvic abscess |
| Scabies (*Sarcoptes scabiei*) | Pruritus. Burrows are fine wavy lines up to 1 cm long | Scrapings from burrows mixed with clear solution (water, KOH, mineral oil); mite seen through microscope | Permethrin cream 5% applied from neck down for 8–14 hours *or* lindane 1% cream, 30 g, thinly applied from neck down for 8 hours *or* sulfur 6% precipitate in ointment applied to entire body nightly on 3 consecutive nights (Medications to be washed off thoroughly after prescribed application) | Thoroughly wash clothing and bedding at high temperature or dry clean. Symptoms result from a sensitivity reaction to the mites |

| | | | | |
|---|---|---|---|---|
| Syphilis (*Treponema pallidum*) | Painless, indurated ulcer at site of exposure; variable rash ("the great imitator"); lymphadenopathy | Spirochetes on darkfield exam; positive serologic test with rising titer (>90 days from lesion onset) | See text | See text |
| Trichomoniasis (*Trichomonas vaginalis*) | Yellow-green vaginal discharge, irritation. | Motile trichomonads on wet mount | Metronidazole 500 mg bid × 7 days *or* 2 g orally as single dose (less effective) | — |

bid = twice a day; HIV = human immunodeficiency virus; HSV = herpes simplex virus; IM = intramuscularly; KOH = potassium hydroxide; PID = pelvic inflammatory disease; qid = four times a day; RPR = rapid plasma reagin

**Source:** From Zakim, D and Boyer, TD: Hepatology: A Textbook of Liver Disease, ed. 2. W. B. Saunders, Philadelphia, 1990, p 895, with permission.

instance, can be transmitted through inanimate objects such as clothing or towels. Hepatitis B and HIV infection can be acquired parenterally through contaminated blood products or needles.

*CONTROVERSY: Even when sexual transmission is thought to be an issue, partners are not always treated. Usually, only the patient is treated for isolated episodes of bacterial vaginosis or condyloma.*

PEARL: With the exception of hepatitis B, none of these diseases results in natural immunity after the first infection, nor have vaccines been developed for them.

## HEPATITIS B

The hepatitis B virus is spherical and consists of three distinctly identifiable proteins or antigens (Fig. 7–1). Of the three hepatitis B proteins, one of them is in the outer coat of the virus and is recognized in blood testing as the hepatitis surface antigen (HBsAG). The coat surrounds an inner protein known as inner core antigen (HBcAG). A third protein, also associated with the inner core, is referred to as hepatitis e antigen (HBeAG). Patients usually become symptom free after the surface antigen has been present in the bloodstream for 3 to 6 weeks. The appearance of e antigen denotes significant liver disease and a highly infectious state. Individuals without evidence of surface antigen and with anticore antibody are only rarely infectious.

The virus may be transmitted through contact with blood or semen from infected persons. Saliva does not appear to be a major route of transmission. Intrauterine infection has been documented, although direct exposure to contaminated maternal bodily fluids is probably a more common route of infection of newborn infants. Both passive and active immunization shortly after birth has been shown to prevent newborn infection.

### Symptoms

Most people acquiring a hepatitis B infection probably remain free of symptoms and develop permanent

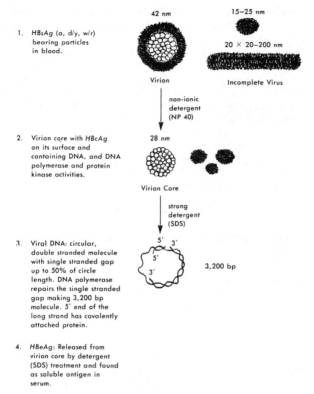

1. *HBsAg (a, d/y, w/r)* bearing particles in blood.

2. Virion core with *HBcAg* on its surface and containing DNA, and DNA polymerase and protein kinase activities.

3. Viral DNA: circular, double stranded molecule with single stranded gap up to 50% of circle length. DNA polymerase repairs the single stranded gap making 3,200 bp molecule. 5' end of the long strand has covalently attached protein.

4. *HBeAg*: Released from virion core by detergent (SDS) treatment and found as soluble antigen in serum.

**Figure 7–1.** Hepatitis B virus. (From Zakim, D and Boyer, TD: Hepatology: A Textbook of Liver Disease, ed 2. W. B. Saunders, Philadelphia, 1990, p 895, with permission.)

immunity. **PEARL: Only 20% of infected individuals develop symptoms of any kind.** The incubation period for symptomatic patients typically lasts from 40 to 110 days but can vary with the number of viral particles initially introduced into the body and the method and site of exposure.

Symptoms consist of a transient illness characterized by fever, malaise, loss of appetite, nausea, and vomiting. They may include a rash consisting of flat, red areas that itch and arthritis that affects the hands and the larger joints of the arms and legs. From 3 to 10 days after onset, the victim begins to turn yellow. As the jaundice worsens over a 2-week period, the patient gradually feels better. The jaundice fades during a 2- to 4-week recovery phase, and a long-lasting immunity to reinfection ensues.

**PEARL: Ten percent of those infected by hepatitis B (approximately half of the symptomatic group) are not able to get rid of surface antigen. These are the people who develop long-term disease.** After developing the temporary type of hepatitis just discussed, these individuals generally show evidence of long-term disease as well.

**PEARL: Some patients simply become asymptomatic long-term carriers of the hepatitis virus. A second subgroup develops persistent hepatitis, with years of mild liver inflammation that eventually resolves. A third subgroup, those with chronic active hepatitis, experience recurrent symptoms of hepatitis for several years.** These individuals are at increased risk for a variety of diseases including cirrhosis and liver cancer. A small fraction of this group die from the disease.

## Diagnosis

The simplest method of diagnosing hepatitis B is by blood studies that test for the various antigens and antibodies (Table 7–2). As mentioned earlier, surface antigen is the first sign of infection, followed by anticore and anti-e antibodies. The appearance of antisurface antibody signals the resolution of infection and suggests long-term immunity to reinfection. Occasionally, a liver biopsy is a necessary diagnostic adjunct to blood testing.

## Prevention and Treatment

Significant advances have been made in recent years to prevent the disease from spreading. Immunizations can take one of two forms: passive and active. Passive immunization involves the injection of antibody directly into the body. It is useful following known ex-

**Table 7–2. SEROLOGIC DIAGNOSIS
OF HEPATITIS B**

| Findings | Significance |
| --- | --- |
| Hepatitis B surface antigen | Patient infectious |
| Hepatitis B surface antibody | Patient immune and not infectious |
| Hepatitis B e antigen | Patient highly infectious; liver disease probable |

posure to infected persons. In contrast, active immunization involves the injection of harmless portions of the hepatitis virus, causing the body to develop its own antibodies. The advantage of active immunization is that the body remains protected for years by its own natural response. Active immunization takes months to work, however, so it is not helpful for recent known exposure.

The hepatitis B vaccine for active immunization was introduced in 1981. It is administered three times over 6 months and is recommended for people at high risk for exposure, such as male homosexuals, prostitutes, dialysis patients, and health care workers. Treatment for an established hepatitis B infection is primarily palliative.

## GENITAL HERPES INFECTION

Genital herpes is caused by the herpes simplex virus (HSV; Fig. 7–2). There are two distinct types of this virus, HSV-1 and HSV-2. Both types are capable of causing genital infections and complications. HSV-1 is most commonly associated with oral "fever blisters," however. Between attacks, it typically remains in a latent state in nerves within the head. On the other hand, HSV-2 resides in the nerves close to the sacrum between recurrences and is most commonly associated with genital infections.

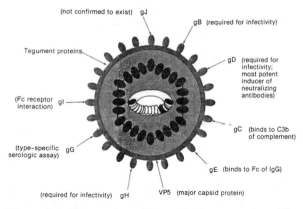

**Figure 7–2.** Herpes virus. (From Whitley, RJ and Middlebrooks, M: Herpes simplex virus infections. In Wyngaarden JB, Smith LH Jr, and Bennett JC [eds]: Cecil Textbook of Medicine, ed. 19. W. B. Saunders, Philadelphia, 1992, p 1831, with permission.)

## Symptoms

The symptoms of the first bout of a genital herpes infection vary greatly. In some, these infections are entirely asymptomatic, but often first-time episodes of genital herpes involve the sudden appearance of small, rapidly spreading, raised sores on the external genitalia. As the illness progresses, these sores combine into large areas of ulceration. Sores persist from 4 to 15 days. Healing is accomplished by crusting and the ingrowth of normal skin, with little residual scarring. New sores can appear for 4 to 10 days after the appearance of the initial one.

These initial episodes tend to be extremely painful and are frequently accompanied by itching, pain on urination, and a vaginal or urethral discharge. By the second week of the illness, the groin lymph nodes become tender; this tenderness is often the last symptom to resolve. Generalized symptoms including fever, headache, malaise, and muscle aches may follow the onset of local sores by 3 to 4 days.

**PEARL: A recurrence of genital herpes infection is usu-**

**ally a much milder illness than the first outbreak, with symptoms limited to the genitalia.** Typically the sores are less painful and less itchy than those of the primary infection, and they resolve after 8 to 12 days. Recurrences are often characterized by the appearance of only one or two sores, which involve less surface area than those in the primary episode.

## Diagnosis

Diagnosis is often clinically based and dependent on observing the characteristic painful vesicles in the genital region. A viral culture can be obtained by unroofing the vesicles with a cotton swab, but if the lesions are already starting to heal, false-negative results become increasingly common.

## Treatment

Therapy for genital herpes is provided in three clinical circumstances: initial infection, recurrences, and prevention (suppression) of recurrences. Medications and dosages for each scenario are summarized in Table 7–3.

## HUMAN IMUNODEFICIENCY VIRUS INFECTION

The human immunodeficiency virus (HIV) is closely related to the human T-cell leukemia virus, the first virus ever to be clearly demonstrated to be a cause of human cancer (leukemia). A retrovirus, HIV has an enzyme, reverse transcriptase, that codes DNA from RNA.

Acquired immunodeficiency syndrome (AIDS), the clinical syndrome caused by HIV, appears to be entirely new to humanity. No illness resembling AIDS was recognized in the United States before 1981. Investigators have speculated that HIV is a mutation of a virus known to infect monkeys in Africa, but the precise origin of this agent remains uncertain. It infects a specific type of lymphocyte (the T-helper cell) and thus renders the body defenseless against normally harmless organisms.

## Table 7–3. TREATMENT OF GENITAL HERPES*

| Medication | For Initial Outbreak | For Recurrent Outbreak | To Suppress Recurrences |
|---|---|---|---|
| Acyclovir (Zovirax) (200, 400, 800 mg) | 200 mg 5 times/day × 10 days | 200 mg 5 times/day × 5 days | 400 mg bid for 1 year |
| Famciclovir (Famvir) (125, 250, 500 mg) | — | 125 mg bid × 5 days | — |
| Valacyclovir (Valtrex) (500 mg, 1000 mg) | 500 mg bid × 10 days | 500 mg bid × 5 days | — |

*Food and Drug Administration (FDA)–approved indications and dosages.

Although homosexual contact and parenteral drug use still account for most new cases in the United States, heterosexual contact is an important route of transmission, particularly for women who may have intercourse unknowingly with high-risk men.

## Symptoms

A person who is infected with HIV commonly remains asymptomatic for months to years. In one study, only 20% of patients remained asymptomatic after 7.5 years of infection. When symptoms develop, they characteristically include severe weight loss, fever, and lymphadenopathy, but they can vary widely depending on which opportunistic infection strikes first. The most common such infection is *Pneumocystis carinii* pneumonia, which occurs in 60% of those with clinically recognized AIDS. With this type of pneumonia, patients complain of shortness of breath and a productive cough for 2 to 4 weeks before they invariably become severely ill and require hospitalization. This pneumonia is differentiated from other severe illnesses by transbronchial lung biopsy.

Perhaps as many as 25% of those who develop AIDS present with a cancer known as Kaposi's sarcoma. Before the arrival of the AIDS virus, this was a slow-growing cancer usually found on the skin of the lower extremity in elderly men of Mediterranean descent. Survival averaged 8 to 13 years, and death usually occurred through the development of a secondary cancer. In those with AIDS, however, Kaposi's sarcoma is much more aggressive and deadly. It consists of reddish purple to dark blue flat or raised sores that first commonly appear on the legs. The lesions may resemble insect bites or bruises, but they often spread over much of the body. Occasionally, the sores can first develop internally in the gastrointestinal tract.

## Diagnosis

The diagnosis of HIV infection is based largely on the laboratory finding of HIV antibody in the patient's serum. It is thought that 95% of those with the virus will have detectable antibody within a few months of becoming infected. Both false-negative and false-positive results are possible on screening; however, the sensitivity and specificity of the test depend directly on the prevalence of the disease in the population being screened. **PEARL: The risk that a positive HIV antibody screen will prove false can be over 50% in a low-risk woman.** As a result, other tests have been developed both to diagnose the infection and follow its course:

- **Serum HIV p24 antigen.** This test can be used to diagnose HIV infection before seroconversion. Paradoxically, as antibody levels go up, immune complexes are formed and p24 antigen levels drop.
- **HIV RNA or branched DNA polymerase chain reaction (PCR).** This test is primarily used to follow the disease course by measuring viral load. Some patients receiving combination antiretroviral therapy actually have no detectable viral genomes in their serum, leading to serious speculation about whether this therapy represents a "cure."
- **CD4+ and CD8+ lymphocyte subsets.** Although HIV affects diverse aspects of the immune system, it seems to have a predilection for CD4 (T4) receptor lymphocytes. CD8 (T8) lymphocytes rebound faster after the initial infection, so the T4/T8 ratio is inverted. **PEARL: Absolute CD4 levels are often used to guide treatment decisions. Cell counts of less than 200 suggest aggressive disease, even in an asymptomatic patient.**

## Treatment

*CONTROVERSY: HIV therapy is advancing so quickly that the large drop in mortality among patients receiving multiple drugs is barely chronicled in the literature.*

The two groups of drugs commonly used are reverse transcriptase inhibitors (RTI) and protease inhibitors (PI). RTIs work by inhibiting the action of viral reverse transcriptase in converting viral RNA into DNA. Examples include zidovudine (ZDV) and azithymidine (AZT). PIs block the action of HIV protease, which is responsible for the cleavage of viral protein precursors. These drugs, such as saquinavir (Invirase) or ritonavir (Norvir) prevent the production of infectious virions.

Although the field is evolving, there appears to be a growing consensus that a prime objective of treatment, even for patients who are asymptomatic, is to eliminate any evidence of the virus from the bloodstream. A growing trend is to use multiple agents and to switch agents if lab markers or opportunistic infections worsen. Drug resistance has proven to be a problem, and strategies are still being developed.

## PELVIC INFLAMMATORY DISEASE

Pelvic inflammatory disease (PID) is a tubal infection that commonly causes varying degrees of abdominal and pelvic pain, often accompanied by low-grade fever. It can also be associated with inflammation and pain around the liver, a so-called perihepatitis also known as Fitz-Hugh-Curtis syndrome. PID can result from either chlamydia or gonorrhea and, under some circumstances, even from bacteria that are part of the normal vaginal flora. Another bacterium, *Mycoplasma hominis*, has been isolated relatively often from fallopian tubes involved in PID. The invading bacteria, particularly gonorrhea and chlamydia, change the local pH and oxygenation status enough to allow normally nonpathogenic bacteria to thrive. As they do so, the environment changes further, typically wiping out the original invaders. **PEARL: PID is a polymicrobial infection whose organisms change over time so that by the time the patient presents with symptoms, it is often difficult to establish its origin.**

### Symptoms

PID can vary from an asymptomatic, silent infection to a life-threatening illness with peritonitis and septic shock. The most common symptom is gradually worsening, dull, lower abdominal pain. The pain is most often on both sides, but it may be confined to one side. Irregular vaginal bleeding is a common accompaniment and suggests a uterine infection. Nearly all patients have a vaginal discharge (usually with pus) on exam, but only half of them actually complain of this on initial presentation. Fever occurs in slightly fewer than one third of patients. Less common symptoms include pain on urination, rectal inflammation, or upper abdominal discomfort. Because the symptoms are so variable, PID often mimics other conditions such as ectopic (tubal) pregnancy and appendicitis.

## Diagnosis

PID is notoriously difficult to diagnose and is misdiagnosed in as many as 35% of patients. Indeed, the only reliable standard is the demonstration of red, inflamed fallopian tubes or a purulent discharge from the end of the tubes at the time of surgery (i.e., laparoscopic diagnosis). In patients with surgically demonstrated tubal infections, only 50% had a pelvic mass noted on physical exam, and 33% had fever. An elevated white blood cell count or sedimentation rate may also suggest the diagnosis, but these, too, are not always abnormal. However, almost all patients with PID have lower abdominal pain and a purulent vaginal discharge in which white cells exceed epithelial cells on microscopic examination of a wet mount. Surgery is not commonly used in the United States for routine confirmation of a diagnosis of PID, but it can be very helpful in distinguishing PID from ectopic pregnancy, appendicitis, and other potentially serious conditions.

## Treatment

For mild infections (minimal pain, no fever or masses on exam), oral antibiotics can be given on an outpatient basis (Table 7–4). Antibiotic treatment is designed to kill a broad spectrum of microbes. Patients with pelvic masses or fever are usually hospitalized to be sure that the fever resolves and the mass (often a pelvic abscess) recedes. In severe cases that do not improve with med-

### Table 7–4. TREATMENT OF PID

| Outpatient | Inpatient |
|---|---|
| Ceftriaxone 250 mg IM and doxycycline 100 mg po bid for 14 days *or* ofloxacin 400 mg po bid for 14 days and either clindamycin 450 mg po qid or metronidazole 500 mg po bid, each for 14 days | Cefoxitin 2 g IVPB every 6 hours and doxycycline 100 mg IVPB every 12 hours* *or* clindamycin 900 mg IVPB every 8 hours and gentamicin 2 mg/kg loading dose, followed by maintenance dose of 1.5 mg/kg every 8 hours; gentamicin peak and trough levels surrounding the third dose† |

*Continue for 48 hours after clinical improvement. Follow up with oral doxycycline bid for a total of 14 days of treatment.
†Continue for 48 hours after clinical improvement. Follow up with either doxycycline 100 mg po bid or clindamycin 450 mg po qid for a total of 12 days of treatment.
IM = intramuscular; po = orally; bid = twice a day; IVPB = intravenous piggyback; qid = four times a day.

ication, surgery is required to remove the infected tissues, because the infection can be fatal. Fortunately, the infection usually responds to antibiotics and surgical removal is rarely necessary. **PEARL: Patients should be hospitalized for peritonitis, high fever, inability to tolerate oral antibiotics, pregnancy, uncertain diagnosis, or suspicion of a pelvic abscess.**

## Complications

The complications of PID relate to scarring and adhesion formation in and around the fallopian tubes. These complications include chronic abdominal pain, infertility, and an increased risk of ectopic pregnancy. After just one mild episode of PID, an estimated 6% of women are infertile because of fallopian tube scarring. After severe episodes, this number rises as high as 30%. Women who have had severe PID also may have a tenfold increase in their risk of a potentially fatal ectopic pregnancy.

# SYPHILIS

Syphilis is caused by *Treponema pallidum, a* very thin, long bacterium that requires a small amount of oxygen to survive. It is so narrow that it is not visible by a conventional microscope, but it can be seen with special techniques (i.e., darkfield exam). Under the microscope, the organism moves with a characteristic corkscrew motion. It does not seem able to penetrate intact skin surfaces but can invade directly through the surfaces that line the mouth, the inside of the penis, the vagina, and the rectum.

## Symptoms

Syphilis symptoms vary greatly depending on the stage of the disease. The first stage, primary syphilis, is marked by the development of a chancre (sore) between 10 and 90 days after inoculation. The chancre occurs at the site of transmission and is therefore commonly found in the genital region, but it can be found anywhere on the body. Because the chancre may be located within the vagina, rectum, or throat, it may not be visible to the patient. Chancres are firm, painless, and smooth but may become covered by a grayish coating. Often, lymph nodes are swollen but not tender. Chancres are not always solitary, as is commonly believed. Secondary infection may make them painful. They start to break down and can lead to painful lymph node swelling. Without treatment, the chancre lasts from 2 to 8 weeks and can occasionally relapse.

The secondary stage of syphilis occurs approximately 6 weeks after the chancre first appears, as the bacteria reproduce and spread through the bloodstream. Besides a variety of skin rashes, the patient often develops fever, malaise, headache, loss of appetite, and swollen lymph nodes. These symptoms are usually mild and temporary. Hepatitis, kidney problems, arthritis, muscle inflammation, and meningitis have all been reported but are not common.

The most prominent symptom of secondary syphilis is the rash. Although the rashes vary widely between individuals, in a given person the rash is generally of one specific type at a particular time and is usually widespread. The rash can resemble numerous other dermatoses. A helpful observation is finding the rash on the palms of the hands and the soles of the feet, because this pattern is characteristic of syphilis and little else in medicine.

Rashes of secondary syphilis heal spontaneously within 2 to 10 weeks. They may leave a residual alteration in skin pigmentation. Without proper treatment, sores may recur up to 4 years after the appearance of the chancre, although recurrence of the rash is rare after 2 years.

Symptoms of the third stage (tertiary syphilis) are discussed in the section on complications.

## Diagnosis

Detection of syphilis is greatly complicated by the different stages of the illness and the myriad symptoms that can accompany each stage. The bacteria can be seen by examining swabbings from the chancre or skin sores, but the usefulness of this technique is limited because the sores shed microbes for only a brief period. As a result, the diagnosis of syphilis has come to rely on a variety of blood tests.

Two serologic tests are typically used. The rapid plasma reagin (RPR) can detect circulating antibodies produced by the body as a reaction to the presence of syphilis. **PEARL: An RPR test will not detect infection until 4 to 6 weeks after initial infection or 1 to 3 weeks after the chancre appears.** The result of the RPR test is almost always positive in secondary syphilis and shows high values. In the late forms of syphilis, the results vary and may not be elevated. Falling levels during treatment of primary or secondary syphilis or stable levels during late syphilis are signs that the therapy is making progress.

An additional test, the fluorescent treponemal antibody test (FTA-ABS), can help confirm a positive RPR result. This test measures the presence and quantity of circulating antibodies that result from an infection with *T. pallidum*. Once positive, this test result rarely if ever becomes negative again, even following treatment.

Unfortunately for the peace of mind of the patient, the RPR may falsely indicate syphilis if some noninfectious diseases, such as lupus, are present. False-positive test results also may occur in the presence of some infectious diseases (e.g., mononucleosis and leprosy) or even in those who are pregnant, elderly, or addicted to drugs. False-positive RPR results typically show low antibody titers and usually can be detected by a negative FTA-ABS.

## Treatment

Syphilis usually responds readily to a variety of antibiotics, which can be administered in several ways, including by mouth (Table 7–5). An unusual reaction can develop within hours after beginning the medication. Known as the Jarisch-Herxheimer reaction, it consists of fever, malaise, headache, nausea, and muscle aches. Skin sores may be intensified or may appear for the first time. The cause is uncertain, but the condition is self-limiting and resolves within a day or so.

### Table 7–5. TREATMENT OF SYPHILIS

| Type of Syphilis | Treatment |
| --- | --- |
| Syphilis of < 1 year duration | Benzathine penicillin 2.4 million units IM *or* doxycycline 100 mg po bid for 14 days |
| Late latent syphilis, > 1 year duration (rule out neurosyphilis with spinal tap) | Benzathine penicillin 2.4 million units IM once a week for 3 weeks *or* doxycycline 100 mg po bid for 4 weeks |
| Neurosyphilis | 2–4 million units aqueous penicillin G IVPB every 4 hours for 10–14 days |

IM = intramuscular; po = orally; bid = twice a day; IVPB = intravenous piggyback.

## Complications

Untreated patients with syphilis often are able to eliminate their infection spontaneously after the second stage and, in some cases, after the appearance of the initial chancre. But even today, one third of those who get syphilis and are not treated will die, developing the serious complications of late syphilis many years following their initial infection.

### *Latent Syphilis*

When patients first contract the disease, they enter an asymptomatic period known as latent syphilis. The World Health Organization (WHO) has divided latent syphilis into two stages, early and late. Early latent syphilis has been further separated according to whether its duration has been less than 1 year or more than 1 year. Patients with a history of chancre and a newly positive blood test result within the past year are considered contagious. Others are still in the early latent stage but are not contagious, except that a pregnant woman in this stage can transmit the infection to her fetus.

When 4 years have passed from the onset of symptoms, the individual is considered to have late latent syphilis, an asymptomatic condition that can last for many years. The diagnosis of this stage relies on a positive blood test result and a history suggesting syphilis. Even without documented treatment, symptoms, or evidence of tertiary syphilis, a positive blood test result is sufficient evidence to diagnose late latent syphilis. These patients require treatment.

### *Tertiary Syphilis*

Symptoms begin to appear again in the late or tertiary stage of syphilis, typically beginning about 5 years after the initial onset. This is the destructive phase of the disease, although patients are noninfectious. It takes five common forms:

- **Mucocutaneous syphilis** usually appears 5 to 20 years after the onset and consists of various types of rashes. All are painless, slow growing, and destructive. They can resolve spontaneously but usually leave a scar. Most commonly, the sores are reddish brown and hard, eventually breaking down the skin in their center.

- **Osseous (bone) syphilis** most often involves the long bones such as the tibia, as well as the skull and the clavicle. The invasion of bone results in local tenderness, structural weakness, and altered shape. For instance, the tibia may develop a thickened anterior surface, causing it to resemble a saber.
- **Visceral syphilis** can cause destruction of the lungs, liver, or stomach through an inflammatory reaction to local accumulation of bacteria from syphilis.
- **Cardiovascular syphilis** results in a weakening of the walls of arteries, particularly the aorta. The result often is heart dysfunction and ultimately heart failure and death.
- **Neurosyphilis** is perhaps the most significant and morbid complication of the disease. The spinal cord and brain are directly invaded by *T. pallidum*. Before antibiotics, a large number of victims were institutionalized. Paralysis and eventual death may also result. The diagnosis of neurosyphilis requires finding characteristic abnormalities in a spinal tap.

### *Congenital Syphilis*

Syphilis poses a grave threat to fetuses. The disease can cause miscarriage or neonatal death. The key to the outlook for the fetus of mothers infected with syphilis is the time that has elapsed since the mother first acquired the infection. Primary and secondary syphilis are well known to present a serious threat to the fetus, and this risk may remain even during the late latent stage of the disease. Children born to women with tertiary syphilis may escape unscathed or may develop a long illness.

For those infants unfortunate enough to be exposed directly to syphilis bacteria from their mother's infection, the consequences can be stillbirth, paralysis, blindness, deafness, and facial abnormalities. Infants born alive who have active skin sores or especially a nasal discharge pose an infectious threat. Syphilis is such a terrible disease for the unborn that it is common practice to screen mothers for the illness as a routine part of prenatal testing.

# 8
## CHAPTER

# *Colposcopy Clinic*

Colposcopy is the examination of vaginal and cervical tissues by means of a magnifying instrument called a colposcope. The procedure is used to select sites of abnormal epithelium for biopsy in patients with abnormal Papanicolaou (Pap) smears.

Cervical cancer kills approximately 4500 women per year in the United States. This figure would be higher were it not for the availability of the Pap smear, although it would probably be lower if more women were tested regularly. It appears that an antecedent infection with the human papillomavirus (HPV) is at least necessary if not sufficient for the development of premalignant and malignant cervical neoplasms.

This chapter reviews the biology of premalignant conditions of the cervix and lower genital tract, particularly as it relates to HPV. New technologies to improve Pap smear accuracy and the follow-up and treatment of abnormal Pap smears is then discussed.

## MICROSCOPIC ANATOMY OF THE CERVIX

The endocervical canal is lined with columnar epithelium that covers a surface with numerous invaginations, the endocervical glands. The columnar cells produce cervical mucus and are directly affected by the cyclic changes in estrogen and progesterone. In contrast to the canal, the cervical portio is covered with squamous epithelium—flat cells, in contrast to the columnar cells. **PEARL: The region where the two types of cells meet is known as the transformation zone because it is here that the columnar cells undergo a process known as metaplasia, whereby they gradually turn into squamous cells. The borders of the transformation zone are the original squamous-columnar junction distally and the new squamous-columnar junction proximally. The transformation zone is critically important because it is here that HPV has been linked to causing cells to transform into neoplasms.**

Typically, the transformation zone tends to move closer to the endocervical canal with age, so that by the time of menopause, the proximal border of this area is actually within the canal. In pregnancy, however, the transformation zone tends to move out toward the portio, at least temporarily. These two separate coverings of the cervix are actually visible under the low-power magnification of the colposcope. A cervix in a young teen that looks quite red typically has a transformation zone far out on the portio, so that the columnar epithelium covers most of the cervix. Years ago we thought this was a pathologic condition called an erosion and treated it, but now we know that it is normal.

Two separate diseases, squamous cell cancer and adenocarcinoma, fall within the category of cervical cancer. The vast majority of cervical cancers are squamous cell in origin, and it is this type of cancer that is thought to result from HPV infection. The less common adenocarcinoma of the cervix arises in the endocervical glands, and its etiology is unclear. Adenocarcinoma is much more difficult to diagnose because it typically remains hidden deep within the endocervical canal.

## HUMAN PAPILLOMAVIRUS

### Principles of Transmission and Management

There is much that we do not yet understand about HPV, although there is growing evidence that the virus is strongly associated with the development of both premalignant conditions and squamous cell cancer of the cervix. HPV also causes condyloma acuminatum (warts) on the vulva and vagina, and it is thought that women with these warts have a lifelong increased risk of developing cancer in these locations. Because these cancers are rare to begin with, however, they are uncommon even among women with a history of condyloma. HPV is known to be spread through sexual intercourse.

*CONTROVERSY: HPV is probably not spread via casual personal contact or contact with contaminated fomites (e.g., towels, toilet seats, doorknobs), but this is not known for sure.*

Among male homosexuals, HPV causes an increase in anal cancer, but otherwise it is not associated with significant morbidity among men. Seventy viral strains have been identified. The strains that cause genital warts are similar to but distinct from those that cause warts on the hands or feet.

Some general principles have emerged from our present knowledge:

- Although HPV DNA can be detected in many women with no evidence of intraepithelial neoplasia, the significance of this finding is not clear. It does not necessarily follow that these women are either contagious or have an increased risk of cervical cancer.
- Although some evidence suggests that some viral strains may be more virulent than others, HPV DNA typing has not proven to be clinically useful to date.

*CONTROVERSY: On the contrary, testing has become so sensitive that it can identify viral DNA in women with normal Pap smears who probably have no meaningful increased risk of developing cervical cancer.*

- The few studies that have evaluated the value of aggressive follow-up of sexual partners have failed to show any consistent benefit.
- Clinical disease, in the form of genital condylomata or cervical dysplasia, is thought to be contagious. The infectiousness of patients with HPV DNA but

without other evidence of disease is not known but is presumably less.

**PEARL: The objective of treatment should be the elimination of symptomatic lesions and the prevention of lower genital tract cancer, not to eradicate all evidence of the viral DNA per se.**

## Treatment of Condylomata

In women, condylomata resulting from HPV infection can appear on three organs: the vulva, the vagina, and the cervix. For vulvar lesions, a variety of topical agents can be applied periodically by the clinician or the patient herself (see Table 7–1). The lesions can also be destroyed with either electrocautery or laser. External condylomata have a relatively high rate of recurrence, but regular treatment eventually eliminates symptoms in most patients. In treating external condylomata, remember that an occasional premalignant or malignant lesion can resemble a simple wart. Although not all condylomata need to be biopsied, women with persistent lesions or particularly stubborn recurrences should probably be investigated more closely with tissue pathology. Women with vulvar intraepithelial neoplasia should probably be treated with laser ablation of the lesions. Also, the vulva should be thoroughly inspected, perhaps under magnification with the colposcope, because these premalignant lesions can occur in more than one area.

Vaginal condylomata can be treated with laser or Efudex 5% cream (5-fluorouracil). Laser treatment tends to be time-consuming, expensive, and incomplete. Efudex is inexpensive and easy to apply, but its dosage and efficacy are not well established. A common regimen is one fourth of an applicator one night per week for 6 weeks. Intercourse should be avoided for 24 hours after the application. Efudex can be highly irritating to vulvar tissues, and treatment should be stopped at the first complaint of perineal pain or burning.

*CONTROVERSY: The benefit of treating small vaginal condylomata has not been clearly established.*

Cervical condylomata can be excised with a cone biopsy or destroyed with cryosurgery or laser. As dis-

cussed later, treatment of uncomplicated cervical condylomata is controversial because many of these lesions
spontaneously resolve over time.

## BIOLOGY OF CERVICAL
## INTRAEPITHELIAL NEOPLASIA

The development of cervical cancer appears to follow
a progression from condyloma to mild dysplasia or cervical intraepithelial neoplasia I (CIN I), to moderate
dysplasia (CIN II), and finally severe dysplasia (CIN III).
The degree of abnormality is determined by how much
of the thickness of the squamous epithelial layer of the
cervix is occupied by immature, abnormal-appearing
cells (Fig. 8–1). CIN I typically involves only the lower

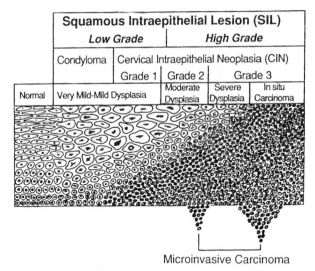

| Squamous Intraepithelial Lesion (SIL) | | | | |
|---|---|---|---|---|
| Low Grade | | High Grade | | |
| Condyloma | Cervical Intraepithelial Neoplasia (CIN) | | | |
| | Grade 1 | Grade 2 | Grade 3 | |
| Normal | Very Mild-Mild Dysplasia | Moderate Dysplasia | Severe Dysplasia | In situ Carcinoma |

Microinvasive Carcinoma

**Figure 8–1.** Cervical squamous carcinoma precursors and the
different terminologies that have been used to refer to them.
The risk of developing microinvasion from the different states
of squamous intraepithelial lesion or different CIN grades is
not necessarily proportional to that illustrated in this drawing.
(From Wright, TC, Kurman, RJ, and Ferenczy, A: Precancer-
ous lesions of the cervix. In Kurman, RJ [ed]: Blaustein's
Pathology of the Female Genital Tract, ed 4. Springer-Verlag
New York, 1994, p 246, with permission.)

third of the epithelium, whereas CIN III involves the entire thickness.

Although the details of this neoplastic process are not fully understood, some general principles seem to emerge. By definition, all premalignant lesions of the cervix can spontaneously regress (or heal) instead of progressing to cancer. Also, the probability that a lesion will progress to a malignancy (as well as the time required for this progression) is directly related to the degree of abnormality. **PEARL: An estimated 1% to 2% of women with mild dysplasia ultimately develop cervical cancer without treatment, whereas the corresponding figure for those with moderate dysplasia is 20% and for those with severe dysplasia is between 30% and 50%. (These are estimates only; there is not a large body of observations of women with these conditions who were followed and not treated.)**

*CONTROVERSY: A current controversy concerns whether or not condylomata and mild dysplasia are actually different entities. A separate debate centers on whether either condition should be treated and how patients with mild dysplasia should be followed if they are not treated.*

The idea that some strains of HPV are particularly oncogenic still seems to have some validity, but the relationship between strain type and prognosis becomes somewhat less clear as more information emerges. It is known that some patients do not undergo an orderly progression from mild to moderate to severe dysplasia and then to cancer; they may skip steps in the progression or go from a normal Pap smear to cancer the next year.

## CERVICAL CYTOLOGY

Developed in 1940 by a Greek American, George Papanicolaou, the Pap smear has proved to be a very successful screening tool for premalignant lesions of the cervix. As a screening tool, a Pap smear alone is not capable of diagnosing a condition; it merely finds patients who require additional investigation and follow-up. **PEARL: A normal Pap smear does not prove that a woman** does not have cervical cancer, nor does an abnormal Pap smear prove that she has condyloma or intraepithelial neoplasia.

## Pap Smear Technique

The cervix needs to be clearly visible for a Pap smear to be performed. Use a Cytobrush (or similar device) to swab the cervical canal. Immediately afterward, apply a wooden spatula to the center of the cervix and rotate it 360 degrees. Within a few seconds, roll the Cytobrush across a portion of the slide and then smear the spatula across the remaining portion. Quickly spray the slide with fixative. The test is very sensitive to air-drying, which causes artifact. Label each Pap slide in pencil with the patient's name and date before it leaves the exam room and before the next patient is brought into the room, to minimize the possibility of mix-ups.

Several new technologies have been introduced in the past few years to address the issue of false-negative Pap smears. Although sampling error has been thought to be the cause of some false-negative results, up to 50% of these errors are attributable to so-called misreading of the material on the slide itself. Two separate computer-based techniques, PapNet and AutoPap 200, have been approved by the Food and Drug Administration (FDA) to rescreen normal smears. A third approach is the Thin Prep, in which the cervix is swabbed in the usual fashion but rather than wiping the swab across a slide and then fixing it, the swab is placed directly into a vial containing preservative. This results in a much higher yield of cells for analysis and simultaneously separates blood cells and mucus from cervical cells, resulting in a less cluttered microscopic image that is easier to read.

*CONTROVERSY: Although the Thin Prep does reduce the rate of false-negative results, it remains controversial because it is four times more expensive and its improved accuracy has not been compared with that of conventional Pap smears rescreened by computer (a less expensive process).*

Most false-negative results represent low-grade lesions; conventional Pap smears missed moderate or severe dysplasia in only 11 patients of 6747 screened in one published study.

## The Bethesda System

Because of the significant false-positive and false-negative rates of Pap smears, there have been ongoing efforts to improve and standardize cytologic reporting. Unfortunately, cytology is inherently a difficult and somewhat subjective process, and some aspects of Pap smear reporting remain controversial. In 1988, at the invitation of the National Institutes of Health, a collection of experts met in Bethesda to agree on a new Pap smear reporting method, and the meeting was reconvened in 1991 to further revise the classification system. The results of these meetings are known as The Bethesda System (TBS). An abbreviated version of TBS is shown in Table 8–1.

## FOLLOW-UP OF ABNORMAL PAP SMEARS

Patients with Pap smears that are satisfactory for evaluation and within normal limits do not require specialized triage. **PEARL: A Pap smear should never be used to diagnose a cervical lesion. Pap smears can be (and have been) interpreted as "normal" in women with grossly visible cervical cancers. Suspicious lesions need to be biopsied.** In this context, it is worth pointing out that normal irregularities and obviously benign lesions appear quite strange to medical students and junior residents. Obtain the advice of an experienced examiner before discussing the need for biopsy with such patients.

If the adequacy of a specimen is given as "satisfactory for evaluation but limited by . . .," specialized follow-up probably is not required if the patient has no recent history of cervical dysplasia. Most patients with unsatisfactory Pap smears should have the smear repeated, but this practice should be individualized.

Patients whose smears show "benign cellular changes"

### Table 8–1. TBS CLASSIFICATION
### OF PAP SMEARS*

I. Adequacy of the Specimen
   A. Satisfactory for evaluation
   B. Satisfactory for evaluation but limited by . . .
   C. Unsatisfactory for evaluation because . . .

II. General Categorization
   A. Within normal limits
   B. Benign cellular changes (see Descriptive Diagnoses)
   C. Epithelial cell abnormality (see Descriptive Diagnoses)

III. Descriptive Diagnoses
   A. Benign cellular changes
      1. Infection (6 subclassifications)
      2. Reactive changes (5 subclassifications)
   B. Epithelial cell abnormalities
      1. Squamous cell
         a. Atypical squamous cells of undetermined significance (describe)
         b. Low-grade squamous intraepithelial lesion (LGSIL); or CIN I (condyloma)
         c. High-grade squamous intraepithelial lesion (HGSIL); or CIN II/III, (carcinoma in situ)
         d. Squamous cell carcinoma
      2. Glandular cell
         a. Endometrial cells, cytologically benign, in postmenopausal woman
         b. Atypical glandular cells of undetermined significance (describe)
         c. Endocervical adenocarcinoma
         d. Endometrial adenocarcinoma
         e. Extrauterine adenocarcinoma
         f. Adenocarcinoma, undetermined source
      3. Other malignant neoplasms
      4. Hormonal evaluation (vaginal smears)

*This classification is abbreviated.

in their general categorization should usually have their Pap smears repeated in 3 to 6 months. Although these Pap smears are not predictive of premalignant changes or subsequent cervical cancer, they are typically more difficult to interpret, and one cannot be as confident that abnormal cells are not hidden. Pap smears may diagnose a specific infection, but using a Pap smear to diagnose an infection is notoriously unreliable.

*CONTROVERSY: Depending on the infectious diagnosis, many clinicians do not treat asymptomatic patients on the basis of the Pap smear; they merely repeat it in several months.*

Patients with glandular cell abnormalities on their Pap smear represent a special problem in diagnosis. The glandular cells are generally hidden from direct view in the cervical canal, and adenocarcinoma with its precursors does not have the same well-defined pattern of progression and treatment protocols as is available for epithelial cell disease. As a result, clinicians tend to follow up even mild glandular cell abnormalities with colposcopy, endocervical curettage (even in the absence of visible lesions) and perhaps an endometrial biopsy at the same time. Endometrial cells seen on a Pap smear in a premenopausal woman have no significance, but after menopause, they require an endometrial biopsy to rule out hyperplasia or malignancy.

*CONTROVERSY: For those with epithelial cell abnormalities, there is debate about whether patients with atypical squamous or glandular cells of undetermined significance should simply receive a follow-up Pap smear in 3 to 6 months or should undergo colposcopy and possible biopsy. The recommendation should be individualized, based largely on the patient's risk factors and the results of her previous Pap smears.*

Malignancies suggested by a Pap smear should be vigorously pursued with biopsy. Low- and high-grade squamous intraepithelial neoplasia should be pursued with colposcopy and biopsy.

Colposcopy is a low-power–magnification examination of the cervix after swabbing away the mucus and discharge with 5% acetic acid (vinegar). The concept behind colposcopy is that dysplasia and squamous cell cancer arise within the transformation zone, and that by carefully examining this biologically active area, one can visually locate and therefore biopsy the most abnormal region. Without the benefit of magnification, randomly performed biopsies of the cervix may miss a premalignant or even malignant lesion.

Premalignant lesions on colposcopy generally appear as some shade of white instead of the normal pink color of the portio or the deeper red of the cervical canal. Some confusion can occur from the normal metaplastic process because columnar epithelium becomes squamous; these areas appear as patchy pale or faint white areas. Generally, brighter white areas, sharp margins, and even raised white areas tend to suggest more severe dysplasia. The pattern of blood vessels in the white area is also used to judge severity: coarse punctation (pin-point vessels) or coarse mosaic (criss-crossing vessels) suggest more serious disease.

*CONTROVERSY: A variety of grading and scoring systems have been proposed for describing colposcopic lesions but the results among different observers vary notoriously.*

The key idea is to biopsy each area that has different features. A colposcopic examination is considered either satisfactory or unsatisfactory. **PEARL: The satisfactory colposcopic exam meets two standards: the entire transformation zone was seen, and all of the borders of any lesion were fully visualized.** If the colposcopy is satisfactory, each different-appearing lesion should be biopsied. As a general rule, an endocervical curettage should also be performed, except in pregnant patients. It is worth noting that patients tend to bleed more with biopsies during pregnancy and that cone biopsies (discussed later) are almost never warranted in pregnant patients.

Any colposcopic exam that does not meet the two standards just mentioned is judged unsatisfactory. In general, patients with dysplasia on a Pap smear and an unsatisfactory colposcopic exam should have a cone biopsy, although it may not be appropriate for those with low-grade lesions. The so-called cone biopsy, in which tissue is removed in the geometric shape of a cone, is intended to remove the entire transformation zone of the cervix, together with a portion of the cervical canal, intact for microscopic evaluation.

# TREATMENT OF SQUAMOUS INTRAEPITHELIAL LESIONS

With TBS, "low-grade squamous intraepithelial lesion" (LGSIL) has replaced the terms "condyloma" and "mild dysplasia"; "high-grade squamous intraepithelial lesion" (HGSIL) is used instead of "moderate dysplasia" and "severe dysplasia" (see Table 8–1).

*CONTROVERSY: The TBS terminology has not been accepted universally, and many cytology labs use both designations to clarify their meanings.*

Five common treatment modalities—cryosurgery, loop electrosurgical excision procedure, laser, cone biopsy, and hysterectomy—exist for squamous intraepithelial neoplasia. All involve physical destruction or removal of the disease tissue.

## Cryosurgery

A specially designed probe is cooled to $-89°C$ with liquid nitrous oxide and then held in place on the cervix for 5 to 10 minutes. The most common protocol calls for a 3-minute freeze, a 2-minute thaw, and another 3-minute freeze. The thaw is achieved by depressurizing the probe, which simply requires depressing the cryo probe trigger further. Efficacy is improved if the freezing is rapid, the ice ball extends at least 5 mm beyond the edge of the probe, and the nitrous oxide tank pressure is kept above 40 kg/cm$^2$. Anesthetics are not typically used, although patients typically experience some degree of menstrual-type cramping. The cramping rapidly dissipates after the procedure and can be minimized with the use of a nonsteroidal anti-inflammatory (such as 600 mg of ibuprofen) taken an hour before the procedure. Destruction of the outer centimeter of the cervix has not been associated with reduced fertility.

## Loop Electrosurgical Excision Procedure

Although there is some argument about semantics, the loop electrosurgical excision procedure (LEEP) is basically a shallow cone biopsy. This procedure is more uncomfortable than cryosurgery, but it has the significant advantage of removing intact tissue for microscopic evaluation. A synonym for LEEP is large loop excision of the transformation zone (LLETZ).

Patient comfort is probably enhanced with local anesthetic, although some physicians do without. The Potacky needle, which has a 20-gauge shaft throughout most of its length but ends in a 27-gauge point, has been specifically developed for this purpose. Typically, 4 mL of 1% lidocaine with epinephrine is injected circumferentially around the cervix. Some physicians also like to administer a paracervical block with a 4-mL injection of 1% lidocaine plain at 3:00 and 9:00 at the base of the cervix after aspirating to be sure that the needle is not in a blood vessel.

The most common loop used is 8 × 20 mm, although many choices exist depending on the patient's cervical anatomy. The current used is typically a blend of cutting and cautery, and the wattage used increases with the size of the electrode, although the settings of the electrosurgical unit vary with the manufacturer. After the patient is grounded and the current is applied, the loop is inserted to a depth of 7 mm or so at one edge of the cervix and swept across the cervical canal. It is then removed straight out at the opposite side of the cervix. The whole process usually takes less than 15 seconds. An effort should be made to move the electrode at a slow, controlled speed. Because this procedure generates a significant smoke plume, a specifically designed speculum and a smoke evacuation unit are necessary.

Some authorities advocate taking an additional portion of the cervix, a sort of core sample, after the first electrode pass. This double-pass procedure removes tissue with a configuration of a cowboy hat. This can be done with a smaller electrode such as 5 × 10-mm loop using lower wattage. Because most lesions are confined to the portio, a double pass may not be necessary for all patients.

In any event, an endocervical curettage should always be performed immediately after LEEP to help ensure that unrecognized disease (even invasive cancer) is not left behind. To prevent subsequent bleeding, the bed of the cervix can be cauterized with a ball electrode and Monsel's solution (ferrous subsulfate) can be applied. The hemisphere of tissue that is removed is often oriented with a suture or india ink to indicate the 12:00 position.

Complications of the procedure include cervical stenosis, which can occur in as many as 3% of patients and generally requires subsequent dilation to remedy. Perhaps 5% of women undergoing the procedure will bleed heavily enough to require medical treatment up to 3 weeks later. This arteriole bleeding generally can be stopped with a reapplication of Monsel's solution, application of hemostatic agents such as Surgicel or Gelfoam, or cervical suturing under sedation, which is rarely needed. The concern about weakening the cervix for future childbearing that may result from a traditional cold-knife cone is generally thought not to be an issue for LEEP procedures, which have a shallower depth of tissue excision.

## Laser

The manufacturer of each $CO_2$ laser usually gives specific instructions, but some general principles can be stated:

- The laser can be used either to destroy cervical tissue, similar to what is done by cryosurgery, or to excise tissue intact for a cone biopsy. For tissue destruction, the cervix is generally lasered to a depth of 7 mm, which can be measured by a calibrated probe. The complications from laser correspond to the type of procedure performed: There are generally none with simple tissue destruction, whereas they resemble those of the LEEP procedure when a cone biopsy is performed.
- Most colposcopes have a focal length of 300 mm. With a laser beam optic focal length of 300 mm, the beam arrives at the surface of the tissue in tight focus, which is ideal for cutting. With the option of a 400-mm focal length optic, the beam is not precisely focused and generally creates a point of destruction in the shape of a hemisphere.
- The power density for cervical tissue cutting or destruction is in the range of 750 to 2000 watts/cm². The corresponding power density for

destruction of vulvar or vaginal lesions is 400 to 600 watts/cm². The actual laser beam width delivered to the tissue needs to be empirically determined through such methods as firing the beam briefly at a tongue depressor and measuring the burn diameter. A laser that delivers 20 watts of power through a 1-mm spot size is actually delivering 2000 watts/cm².

- During the procedure, a specifically designed (i.e., blackened) speculum is needed, together with a smoke evacuation system.
- As with a LEEP, patient comfort is enhanced with local anesthetic and the cervical bed should be treated with Monsel's solution to reduce bleeding after the procedure.

Laser procedures are typically much more expensive and take longer to perform than the available alternatives. With no documented improved efficacy, this approach should generally be reserved for special circumstances such as the destruction of well-defined vaginal or vulvar lesions.

## Cone Biopsy

**PEARL: The cone biopsy can be used for both diagnosis and treatment, and is intended to remove the entire transformation zone intact for histologic examination.** Treatment efficacy can be confirmed by inspecting the surgical margins and confirming that the lesion was entirely removed. A cone biopsy can be carried out with a knife and suture, laser, or LEEP. An endocervical curettage is advisable after a cone biopsy to provide additional information should the lesion extend to the endocervical margin.

Regardless of the method used to perform the cone biopsy, perhaps as many as 5% of patients experience enough bleeding to require medical attention for up to 3 weeks after the procedure. In most cases, the bleeding can be controlled simply by applying Monsel's solution (ferrous subsulfate) to the cervical bed. Bleeding that does not respond to this treatment can be controlled by suturing, although this procedure usually requires general anesthesia. Other complications of cone biopsy include cervical stenosis and cervical incompetence for subsequent pregnancies.

*CONTROVERSY: Cervical incompetence is said to occur 1% of the time after cone biopsies, although this statistic seems somewhat speculative and this probably does not apply to the shallow cone biopsies done as a LEEP.*

## Hysterectomy

This treatment is a consideration only for women who have completed their families. In general, it is appropriate for those who have severe dysplasia by biopsy, positive endocervical curettages, or disease extending to the endocervical resection margin on cone biopsies. To minimize the chance of operative-site infections, hysterectomies are generally delayed until at least 6 weeks after a cone biopsy.

# 9

CHAPTER

# *The Menopause Clinic*

**PEARL: Menopause occurs with the cessation of ovarian function and may be diagnosed after periods have ceased for 1 year. The average age in the United States for menopause is 51.** Before the menopause, menstrual periods typically become infrequent, although they can cease suddenly without warning. It is not uncommon to have some aspect of irregular, frequent bleeding also. Unfortunately, this sort of bleeding can also be a sign of endometrial cancer, the incidence of which rises for women in their early 50s. Women who have abnormal vaginal bleeding (episodes occurring more frequently than every 21 days or lasting longer than 7 days) on two separate occasions in 6 months should have an endometrial biopsy. This is an office procedure done to screen for endometrial malignancy or premalignancy.

Among women undergoing the menopause, 85% will experience "hot flashes"; some never do. The blood test to determine if someone is in the menopause is a follicle-stimulating hormone (FSH) level, which invariably rises in the absence of ovarian production of estrogen. Measuring the estrogen level is not appropriate in this context, as it can vary widely in premenopausal women. An FSH above 50 mIU/mL essentially proves the menopause.

## HORMONE REPLACEMENT THERAPY

Three classes of hormones are relevant to hormone replacement therapy (HRT) in the menopause: estrogens, progestins, and androgens. Estrogen supplementation relieves hot flashes within 7 days. It also prevents vaginal atrophy.

*CONTROVERSY: Some suggest that estrogen supplementation aids in urinary continence by thickening the urethral mucosa. The limited number of studies have not been consistent on this point.*

The estrogen products used for HRT are either naturally occurring or synthetically produced natural estrogens, in contrast to oral contraceptives, which use potent synthetic estrogens. Too much estrogen leads to nausea and breast tenderness, but these side effects are almost never seen with HRT in the menopause. Some studies have also linked estrogen supplementation with increased risk of some types of cancer, as discussed in the next section of this chapter.

Progestin supplementation has very few side effects, although some women may complain of cyclic moodiness or headaches when the 10-mg dose is administered cyclically.

Androgen replacement in the menopause is less universally accepted. It does seem to have some merit, because the ovaries do produce measurable amounts of testosterone during the reproductive years. Unwanted hair growth is a potential disadvantage but is rarely seen with common replacement doses of androgen.

*CONTROVERSY: A few medical studies suggest that testosterone supplementation increases libido and the general sense of well-being, and reduces the amount of estrogen required to control hot flashes.*

A new class of compounds recently has been recognized as having value in HRT. Known as selective estrogen receptor modulators, or SERMs, these drugs have some of the benefits of estrogen but apparently without the cancer-causing potential. The effectiveness of raloxifene (Evista), one of these compounds, in preventing osteoporosis has been well established. It may also provide some protection against heart disease.

## Disease-Preventive Effects of Hormone Replacement Therapy

An issue just as important as relief of menopausal symptoms is the prevention of disease. Table 9–1 shows the estimated effects of various HRT regimens on the annual death rate for women. The key issues that are still being defined include:

- When should HRT be started and how long should it be continued? The general consensus is that hormone replacement should begin within a year or two of the menopause, because an increasing rate of bone loss and heart disease seems to begin at this point. Because the protective benefits cease when the medication is stopped, many believe that it should be continued indefinitely.
- Does estrogen increase the risk of breast cancer (even modestly)? It is clear that any effect on breast cancer is much less pronounced than the increased risk of uterine cancer. Although the bulk of the evidence suggests no increase in risk, it is much more difficult to establish conclusively that a modest risk does not exist. One recent large prospective study did in fact suggest a 30% increase—that is, a change in the risk of breast cancer from about 9% to 12%, not an absolute risk of 30%.
- Does progestin:
  - Reduce the cardiac benefits of concomitant estrogen administration?
  - Affect breast cancer risk?
  - Reduce osteoporosis risk?
- What effect does raloxifene have on heart disease and breast cancer? Preliminary evidence is favorable but not conclusive.
- Does testosterone have a deleterious effect on heart disease? Preliminary, inconclusive evidence suggests that clinically acceptable doses do not have a deleterious effect on heart disease.

Many authorities suggest prescribing the minimum dose of estrogen necessary to alleviate menopausal

**Table 9–1. ANNUAL DEATH RATES FOR WOMEN IN THE UNITED STATES**

| Disease | Natural Incidence | Receiving Estrogen | Receiving Progestin | Receiving Both Hormones | Receiving Raloxifene (Evista) |
|---------|-------------------|--------------------|--------------------|------------------------|-------------------------------|
| Osteoporosis | 15,000 | 75% reduction | Additional reduction? | > 75% reduction? | 75% reduction |
| Heart disease | 250,000 | 50% reduction | Detrimental to cholesterol metabolism and cardiac risk? | Net benefit—degree uncertain | Improved cholesterol metabolism and reduction in cardiac risk? Trials under way |
| Breast cancer | 41,000 | No increased risk to 30% increase? | No effect to reduction in risk? | No increased risk? | Large (up to 50%) reduction in risk? Major trial under way |
| Uterine cancer | 4000 | 400%–800% increased risk | Large reduction in risk | Large reduction in risk | No increased risk |

symptoms or prevent osteoporosis. Although this would appear to be common sense, most of the studies showing the benefits of HRT also show a dose-related benefit—the higher the dose, the greater the reduction in osteoporosis and heart disease.

## Common HRT Regimens

- **Daily administration of an estrogen together with a progestin.** (Example: conjugated estrogens 0.625 mg with medroxyprogesterone acetate 2.5 mg daily.) The objective is to eliminate vaginal bleeding entirely. The drawback is that many women have unpredictable bleeding for the first 6 to 9 months.
- **Cyclic estrogen and progestin.** The estrogen is administered on days 1 to 25 of the calendar month and the progestin (e.g., medroxyprogesterone acetate 10 mg) is given for the last 10 to 14 days (i.e., days 14 to 25). The disadvantage of this regimen is that most patients experience cyclic bleeding at the end of each month for years after menopause.
- **Continuous estrogen and cyclic progestin.** The estrogen is given throughout the cycle, but the progestin is again given for only 10 to 14 days. In theory, since the patient has no estrogen withdrawal, she is less likely to have cyclic bleeding. Premphase is a branded package of pills in which the estrogen and progestin are combined during the second half of the cycle.
- **Raloxifene (Evista)—selective estrogen receptor modulator.** Known in the lay press as "designer estrogen," raloxifene 60 mg can be given once daily without a progestin and without causing withdrawal or breakthrough bleeding. It is not effective against hot flashes or vaginal atrophy, and its role in menopause is still being defined.

## Specific Hormonal Preparations

Table 9–2 lists a wide variety of products (in various forms) that are available for use in HRT. This table does not include the SERM raloxifene (Evista), used in a

## Table 9-2. PRESCRIPTION HORMONE REPLACEMENT THERAPY PRODUCTS

*Oral Estrogens*

**Premarin** (conjugated estrogens) 0.3, 0.625, 0.9, 1.25, 2.5 mg
**Estratab** (conjugated estrogens) 0.3, 0.625, 0.9, 1.25, 2.5 mg
**Ogen** (estropipate) 0.625 (actually 0.75 mg of drug), 1.25 (actually 1.5 mg of drug)
**Ortho-Est** (estropipate) 0.625 mg (actually 0.75 mg of drug), 1.25 mg (actually 1.5 mg of drug)
**Estrace** (estradiol) 0.5, 1.0, 2.0 mg

*Transdermal Estrogens\**

**Alora** (estradiol) 0.05 mg, 0.75 mg, 0.1 mg (nominal daily dose). Twice weekly dosing.
**Climara** (estradiol) 0.05 mg, 0.1 mg (nominal daily dose). Once weekly dosing.
**Estraderm** (estradiol) 0.05 mg, 0.1 mg (nominal daily dose). Twice weekly dosing.
**FemPatch** (estradiol) 0.025 mg (nominal daily dose). Once weekly dosing.
**Vivelle** (estradiol) 0.0375 mg, 0.05 mg, 0.75 mg, 0.1 mg (nominal daily dose). Twice weekly dosing.

*Vaginal Estrogens*

**Premarin Vaginal Cream** (conjugated estrogens) 42.5-g tube. Applicator calibrated to 2 g in ½-g doses.
**Ogen Vaginal Cream** (estropipate) 42.5-g tube with 1-, 2-, 3-, 4-g applicator.
**Estring** (estradiol) 2 mg (nominal daily dose). 90-day vaginal insert.

*Progestins*

**Provera** (medroxyprogesterone acetate) 2.5, 5, 10 mg
**Prometrium** (progesterone) 100 mg
**Crinone** (progesterone cream) 0.4%, 0.8% (use in HRT is "off-label" use).

*Combination Preparations*

**Estratest** (conjugated estrogens, methyltestosterone): Full strength: 1.25 mg/2.5 mg; Half-strength: 0.625 mg/1.25 mg
**Prempro** (conjugated estrogens/medroxyprogesterone acetate): 0.625 mg/2.5 mg, 0.625 mg/5 mg
**Premphase** (conjugated estrogens): 14 days of 0.625 conjugated estrogens, 14 days of 0.625 conjugated estrogens with 5 mg of medroxyprogesterone acetate
**Combi-patch\*** (estradiol/norethindrone acetate): 0.05/0.14, 0.05/0.25 (nominal daily dose in mg)

---

\*Patches can be applied on the abdomen or buttocks but not the hips (where clothing will rub against them) or the breasts (which are sensitive to estrogen).

dose of 60 mg daily (no progestin needed). Many of the preparations shown on the table do have generic equivalents. At this time, there is no separate, branded testosterone for HRT.

Establishing dose equivalency among brands of different estrogens is problematic because the individual hormones have different potencies. With this caveat, Premarin 0.625 mg, Ogen 0.625 (not mg), Estraderm 0.05, and Estrace 1 mg are all roughly equivalent.

Follow-up of a patient who receives a prescription for HRT consists of a return visit at 3 months to see how she is faring and to adjust the dosage or regimen as necessary. Subsequent exams can be performed annually. Contraindications to HRT include a current or recent deep venous thrombosis, active gallbladder or liver disease, or a history of hormone-sensitive cancers such as breast and uterine cancer.

*CONTROVERSY: Some authorities recommend a routine liver function profile before starting treatment, but this seems somewhat zealous for the general population with no history of liver disease.*

As the benefits of estrogen become increasingly clear, the risks of hormone replacement in specific situations are being re-evaluated. It is difficult to make a blanket recommendation, and the treatment decision is usually individualized based on the patient's age, general health, type and stage of cancer (if any), and menopausal symptoms.

*CONTROVERSY: Clinical practice has been changing. It is a growing practice to give hormones to women who have a recent history of an early endometrial cancer if they are free of disease after some arbitrary period of time (6 months to 5 years).*

## OSTEOPOROSIS

**PEARL: As can be seen from Table 9–1, the mortality rate from heart disease for women is almost 17 times higher than that from osteoporosis.** But aside from absolute longevity, we should consider the time of independent living. Given the morbidity from spine, wrist, and hip fractures, eliminating osteoporosis becomes important beyond just lowering the mortality rate.

Osteoporosis occurs when, during the lifelong process of bone remodeling, bone resorption exceeds the rate of bone formation. **PEARL: Present in all ethnic groups and both genders but most common in white women, osteoporosis has been defined by the World Health Organization as a bone mineral density (BMD) 2.5 or more standard deviations below that of a "young, normal" woman.** Osteopenia, or low bone mass, is diagnosed when the BMD is between 1 and 2.5 standard deviations below normal.

Various methods can be used to determine bone density, measuring different sites such as the wrist, hip, spine, or heel. Hip BMD seems to be the best predictor both of hip fractures and fractures at other sites. Because the hip is part of the axial skeleton and is surrounded by widely varying amounts of soft tissue, dual energy photon absorptiometry has proven to be the most useful method of assessing this value. With this technique, photons from two different energy sources are used so that the amount of energy absorbed by the soft tissues can be assessed, leaving a true picture of bone density.

Although the role of estrogen in maintaining bone density has yet to be fully explained, it is clear that cessation of ovarian function causes accelerated bone loss. Early menopause, either from surgical castration or premature ovarian failure, has been linked to a particularly severe loss of bone density. Other risk factors include the use of cigarettes, alcohol, long-term heparin, glucocorticoids, and anticonvulsants. Secondary osteoporosis results from disorders involving calcium metabolism, such as thyrotoxicosis, diabetes, and parathyroid disease.

*CONTROVERSY: Who should get bone density measurements? The National Osteoporosis Foundation suggests that all women 65 and older should be screened, along with younger postmenopausal women who have other risk factors and those presenting with fractures.*

**PEARL: Estrogen replacement therapy is highly effective in preventing osteoporosis and is probably of some benefit**

**in actual treatment.** Progestins and testosterone also may help to restore bone density, but there are less data than for estrogen.

**PEARL: For patients who have osteoporosis despite HRT or those for whom HRT is contraindicated, a separate class of drugs known as bisphosphonates is known to inhibit bone resorption. The first drug approved by the FDA for this purpose is alendronate (Fosamax).** To prevent osteoporosis, 5 mg daily is recommended; 10 mg is preferred to treat established disease. The drug is associated with significant gastrointestinal upset such as heartburn and must be taken on an empty stomach 30 minutes before eating. Heartburn is minimized if the patient remains upright after taking the medication. Nasal calcitonin, 200 mg per day, is also helpful but appears less potent than alendronate.

There is no standard for follow-up studies for those under treatment, but there is probably little value in retesting sooner than a year.

## ASSESSMENT OF POSTMENOPAUSAL BLEEDING

As noted earlier, patients with repeated bleeding episodes lasting longer than 7 days or occurring more frequently than every 21 days need to have some evaluation of their endometrium. Although it is more common for menstrual periods to become lighter and farther apart, many women have more frequent or longer bleeding episodes as the endometrium atrophies. The initiation of HRT also can result in such bleeding patterns. The clinical problem that such patients present is that this type of bleeding can be a presenting symptom of endometrial hyperplasia or neoplasia.

In general, three methods can be used to assess the endometrium: endometrial biopsy, ultrasound, and dilation and curettage (D&C) with hysteroscopy. Because the first two are office procedures, they are typically preferred. To perform an endometrial biopsy, first perform a bimanual exam to determine the orientation of the uterus. Then expose the cervix with a speculum and swab it with iodine. Then place a thin, special-purpose catheter (typically 3 mm or less) through the cervical canal and advance it very gently until the resistance of the top of the uterus is encountered. Apply suction, and then remove the instruments. Record the depth of the uterus, and subjectively assess the amount of tissue obtained. Occasionally, to provide better traction, a single-tooth tenaculum can be used to grasp the anterior lip of the cervix and hold it in place. The procedure typically can be completed within 90 seconds and entails minimal discomfort (i.e., menstrual-type cramping during the procedure).

*CONTROVERSY: One problem that often arises is that the pathology lab will report "insufficient tissue for diagnosis." Because a substantial percentage of the patients undergoing endometrial biopsy have abnormal bleeding due to uterine atrophy, a finding of "insufficient tissue" does not usually warrant further testing unless the abnormal bleeding is quite persistent or becomes heavier.*

Occasionally, an endometrial biopsy cannot be completed, owing to either patient discomfort or peculiarities of anatomy, such as cervical stenosis. In this event, an ultrasound exam can be used to assess the thickness of the uterine lining. **PEARL: In general, an endometrial thickness of 5 mm or less greatly reduces the possibility of hyperplasia or malignancy.** If the endometrium is thickened, a fractional D&C with hysteroscopy under sedation may be necessary.

## PREMATURE OVARIAN FAILURE

**PEARL: The cessation of menstruation before the age of 40 associated with a high FSH level is not menopause but rather premature ovarian failure. This is thought to be an autoimmune process and not the result of natural aging.** Women with premature ovarian failure are sterile and experience a significantly increased risk of heart disease and osteoporosis unless they receive HRT. Because of its autoimmune origin and the concern that other endocrine organs may be at risk, check a fasting morning cortisol level, comprehensive chemistry (for glucose and calcium), two postprandial glucose measurements, thyroid function, and antithyroid antibodies.

# 10
## CHAPTER

# *Reproductive Endocrinology Clinic*

Of couples having unprotected intercourse two times a week or more, 80% to 90% can expect to conceive within 1 year. Approximately 10% suffer from either subfertility or infertility. **PEARL: Thus, an infertile couple is traditionally defined as a couple that fails to conceive within 1 year from the onset of regular sexual intercourse.**

An alternative definition is frequently more useful. This definition regards two people as having a fertility problem if they think they do. The average time to first conception is 5 months. For a healthy man and woman in their 20s who are worried about their inability to conceive after 6 months, all that might be necessary is reassurance. If this same couple were in their late 30s, however, a diagnostic workup might be in order to speed identification of a problem if one exists. Therefore, the traditional 1-year definition of infertility is often flawed. Both hypothetical couples could benefit from acknowledgment of their problem, even if they require only reassurance. Another issue is the fact that the success rate of assisted reproductive technologies drops noticeably as women age, particularly after the age of 40. Therefore, waiting a full year for older couples could reduce the probability of successful treatment should a problem be found.

## EVALUATION OF THE INFERTILE COUPLE

In approximately 40% of infertile couples, the primary problem is related to the male. Characteristically, his sperm count is low or the sperm are in some way abnormal. In contrast, women have two major causes of infertility: (1) anovulation or (2) problems with the reproductive tract itself (tubal obstruction, abnormal uterine anatomy, and so on). Each problem accounts for approximately 40% of female infertility. In a few couples, no cause of infertility is ever found. Occasionally, couples become pregnant for no apparent reason after years of trying.

Protocols vary widely among infertility centers and there is no standardized approach to the workup. In general, though, some sort of screening procedure is done first to assess which of the three areas described earlier is likely to be the source of the problem.

### Semen Quality

The semen analysis is a rather crude indication of a man's fertility. In men with established fertility, semen characteristics and content vary widely both between different men and between samples obtained from the same individual at different times. As a result, the diagnosis of abnormal semen requires at least two abnormal samples. The sample should be obtained after at least 48 hours of abstinence and should arrive at the lab within an hour of collection. Table 10–1 shows characteristics of normal semen.

### Assessment of Ovulation

**PEARL: The commonly used diagnostic tests can only predict that normal ovulation has taken place perhaps 80% of the time.** Unless the egg can be seen directly out-

## Table 10–1. SEMEN ANALYSIS:
## NORMAL CHARACTERISTICS

| | |
|---|---|
| Volume | > 2 mL |
| Count | >20 million/mL |
| Motility | >50% |
| Morphology | >60% oval |
| White cells | Rare, <1 million/mL |

side of the ovary (which is not currently possible), or unless conception has taken place, tests of ovulation are necessarily indirect and flawed.

- **Basal body temperature.** Taken immediately on awakening and at the same time each day, the basal body temperature (BBT) curve will show a rise of approximately 0.4° F for no less than 11 days in most ovulatory cycles. Of course, the test is not perfectly accurate; it can miss some who ovulate and misidentify some who did not ovulate.
- **Urinary luteinizing hormone (LH) surge.** Kits intended for home use typically come with five reagent strips per package to test for the surge of LH, which is thought to occur 12 to 24 hours before ovulation.
- **Progesterone level.** Some authorities consider a level of progesterone of 10 ng/mL in the middle of the luteal phase to be suggestive of normal ovulation; others are more comfortable with a level of at least 15 ng/mL. Typically the progesterone level should be measured 5 to 7 days before the first day of the next period.
- **Endometrial biopsy.** An endometrial biopsy involves a gentle sampling of the lining of the uterus 2 to 3 days before the expected menstrual period. The biopsy is typically performed in the office without medication. An occasional patient will experience several minutes of cramping, but the test usually causes minimal discomfort. The pathology examination will typically identify the endometrial lining as proliferative (no recent ovulation) or secretory (recent ovulation). The actual dating of the cycle can be done based on characteristic changes

in the endometrial glands and stroma. Successful ovulation associated with a difference of more than 2 days in the relative rates of maturation of the endometrial glands and the underlying, supporting stromal tissue suggests suboptimal levels of progesterone production following ovulation (so-called luteal phase defect). It is thought that a decrease in total progesterone production may lead to failed implantation or death of the embryo shortly after implantation. This decrease can be treated with either Clomid or progesterone vaginal suppositories (25 mg twice a day after ovulation and through the first trimester of pregnancy).

An endometrial biopsy theoretically can damage or remove the pregnancy if it is performed in a location where a fertilized egg has implanted. In practice, the risk is rather small; there are many reports in the medical literature of pregnancies going to full term even when a biopsy was done (unknowingly) during an early pregnancy. Performing a urine pregnancy test before doing the procedure for infertility is probably a good idea, even though if conception took place within the previous 10 days the test will fail to show it.

- **Serial ultrasonography.** Ultrasound exams that show progressive growth of the largest follicle to at least 18 mm, followed by a sudden collapse, are strongly suggestive of ovulation.
- **Vaginal electrical resistance.** Vaginal electrical resistance has been shown to drop noticeably with the LH surge. This test is used less commonly than the others.

## Assessment of the Female Genital Tract

### *Hysterosalpingogram*

The hysterosalpingogram (HSG) is an x-ray exam of the uterus and fallopian tubes. In this diagnostic test, a small tube is inserted through the cervix and into the uterus. Contrast medium is then pushed into the tube. Several x-ray films are taken as the dye makes its way through the uterus and out into the fallopian tubes. The test helps identify abnormalities within the uterus, as well as any scarring or blockage of the tubes.

Occasionally, the fallopian tubes appear to be blocked when they are not. This appearance can result from tubal "spasm" in which the muscles of the tube contract in response to the test itself. As discussed later, laparoscopy can often resolve this issue if the tubes appear to be blocked.

An HSG actually takes about 15 minutes. Because the test can sometimes be uncomfortable, many prescribe antiprostaglandins an hour or so before performing the study. The HSG can cause a tubal infection or exacerbate an existing infection in a small percentage of patients.

*CONTROVERSY: To reduce the chance of tubal infection, patients are often treated with antibiotics for several days before and after a hysterosalpingogram (e.g., doxycycline 100 mg orally twice daily for 5 days, beginning 2 days before the test).*

### Postcoital Test

A postcoital test involves examining the mucus in the cervical canal 2 hours or so after a couple has had intercourse. The best time for this test is 1 to 3 days before ovulation (or the rise in the basal body temperature), which can be determined by the basal body temperature pattern in previous menstrual cycles. A normal postcoital test result should show five or more moving sperm per field when examined under the microscope. The mucus itself should be able to be stretched to at least 8 cm or so. An abnormal result can suggest problems in either the mucus or the sperm. Recently, the test has become controversial because there is no clear-cut proven benefit from acting on its results. The most common reason for an abnormal postcoital test result is improper timing in the menstrual cycle. Immotile sperm in the presence of favorable mucus may suggest sperm antibodies or a local infection. For this reason, antibiotics (typically doxycycline) are prescribed for those with an abnormal postcoital test result.

*CONTROVERSY: The treatment for sperm antibodies in the serum of either the man or the woman has yet to be firmly established. Alternatives include the use of a condom for several months to reduce semen exposure for the woman, or steroids for the person with elevated levels of sperm antibodies.*

Mucus that is sparse or that immobilizes sperm can be treated with follicular phase estrogens for 8 to 9 days preceding ovulation.

### *Laparoscopy and Hysteroscopy*

*CONTROVERSY: The role of laparoscopy and hysteroscopy in the infertility workup is somewhat controversial. Some authorities advocate early visualization of the peritoneal and uterine cavities, but others suggest the procedure only for those with unexplained infertility.*

## Looking for Endocrinopathies

Occasionally, some infertile women have elevated androgens, suggested by the clinical findings of hirsutism or oily skin (see Hirsutism in Chapter 4). Those with elevated androgens not produced by a neoplasm may benefit from adrenal suppression with corticosteroids such as dexamethasone.

## TREATMENT OF INFERTILITY

One of the problems in assessing treatment efficacy is that the background rate of spontaneously occurring conceptions in the infertile population is significant.

*CONTROVERSY: Few infertility therapies have been subjected to rigorous randomized, prospective studies.*

Nonetheless, there is no doubt that the development of techniques for ovulation induction and the assisted reproductive technologies have resulted in conceptions that would not have taken place otherwise.

## Male Infertility

Three treatment approaches are generally available when semen quality is a problem: improvement of semen quality, improvement of sperm delivery, and the use of donor sperm.

### *Improving Semen Quality*

Additional testing is usually required. One initial step can be to stop tobacco use, which has been linked to a decrease in semen quality. Levels of prolactin and TSH should be checked, because, as in women, abnormalities can interfere with hypothalamic function and cause low levels of pituitary gonadotropins, resulting in low sperm counts or poor motility. Direct treatment of the pituitary or thyroid problem can restore fertility.

Low levels of LH and follicle-stimulating hormone (FSH) can be treated with gonadotropin injections, although a markedly elevated FSH suggests direct damage to testicular tissue.

*CONTROVERSY: A varicosity of the spermatic veins, called a varicocele, is thought to interfere with sperm quality by slightly raising testicular temperature. Ligation of the spermatic vein has been suggested to be beneficial, but evidence of efficacy is weak.*

### *Efforts to Improve Sperm Delivery*

Artificial insemination or even in vitro fertilization can be used when sperm quantity or quality is poor. Both techniques can deliver a higher number of spermatocytes to the vicinity of the ovum than would occur naturally. With artificial insemination, the sperm are often washed to minimize uterine cramping and placed into the uterus during the LH surge, often during a stimulated cycle.

### *Donor Sperm*

In irremediable cases of male infertility, artificial insemination can be done with donor sperm. Sperm donors are screened carefully for sexually transmitted diseases (including acquired immunodeficiency syndrome [AIDS]) and make their contribution anonymously. Sperm donor and recipient never meet, and their identities are carefully guarded.

## Anovulation

Elevated prolactin or abnormal thyroid function in the woman would normally be treated before undertaking more aggressive therapy.

### *Clomiphene Citrate*

A weak estrogen, clomiphene citrate binds to hypothalamic estrogen receptors and results in increased secretion of gonadotropin-releasing hormone (GnRH). This increase in GnRH, in turn, results in a rise in LH and FSH. The medication is typically given for 5 days early in the cycle, typically days 3 through 7 or 5 through 9. Started at 50 mg, the dose is steadily increased in each successive cycle until ovulation is established. Some method of evaluating ovulation is desired, typically a progesterone level 13 to 15 days after the last tablet. The maximum effective and safe dose is variously described but is typically no more than 250 mg; many authorities do not exceed a daily dose of 200 mg.

*CONTROVERSY: For those who do not experience ovulation at higher doses, some have advocated the use of a single intramuscular dose of 10,000 mIU of human chorionic gonadotropin (hCG) 7 days after the last clomiphene tablet, but this approach is controversial. The hormone's similarity to LH is thought to help with the final stages of ovulation.*

**PEARL: Because 80% of conceptions that occur while the patients are on clomiphene occur within three ovulatory cycles, the treatment plan should be re-evaluated if the patient has not conceived after three cycles.** Typical side effects of clomiphene include hot flashes, bloating, breast tenderness, and nausea. The multiple gestation rate is roughly 6% to 8% but very few pregnancies result in more than twins. Ovarian enlargement presenting as significant pelvic pain can be an uncommon complication, but it usually resolves spontaneously with reduced activity.

### *Gonadotropin Treatment*

One of two agents, either human menopausal gonadotropin (a mixture of LH and FSH obtained from the urine of menopausal women) or purified FSH is typically administered intramuscularly on a daily basis beginning between cycle days 2 and 5. Monitoring consists of daily ultrasound assessment of follicle size and number, together with measurement of estradiol levels. As treatment continues, the dosage is adjusted based on follicle development and estrogen levels. When the largest follicle achieves a diameter of 20 mm, 10,000 units of hCG are administered to achieve ovulation. hCG is generally withheld if estradiol levels exceed 2000 pcg/mL owing to the risk of hyperstimulation, although the risk can be more precisely assessed in combination with ultrasound monitoring. The risk of multiple gestations with gonadotropins can range from a low of 5% with low doses to as high as 20% in some series, and more than two fetuses are not uncommon. Hyperstimulation also can produce more serious complications including significant ascites and pleural effusions.

## Female Genital Tract Abnormalities

Tubal obstruction is the classic indication for in vitro fertilization (IVF), although surgical procedures occasionally can be helpful. The pregnancy rate following microsurgical repair of the fallopian tubes varies with the procedure and the anatomy. Tubal ligation reversals have the highest success rate, on the order of 60%. An important complication following tubal surgery is ectopic pregnancy, which can occur in up to 10% of cases.

The treatment of intrauterine lesions such as fibroids and septa is more controversial. As a rule, it is believed that these anatomic abnormalities have to be very significant before they will interfere with fertility. Uterine fibroids and septa are more often suspected of having a role in miscarriage, rather than causing infertility per se.

IVF typically involves a stimulated cycle followed by several further steps:

1. **Oocyte retrieval.** The oocyte must be obtained directly from the ovary. This is not as difficult as it sounds because oocytes are contained within follicles that are easily visible and 2 to 4 cm in diameter. A needle is gently inserted into the follicle, and the fluid with the oocyte floating in it is sucked out. It is then carefully rushed to the laboratory, where it undergoes maturation. The usual approach to retrieval is to use ultrasound to guide a small needle through the back of the vagina directly into the ovarian follicles.

2. **Oocyte maturation.** Most oocytes are not quite ready for fertilization immediately on retrieval. They undergo a somewhat mysterious maturation process for a day or so in the laboratory before they are ready for penetration by sperm.

3. **Fertilization.** If the IVF is being performed because of male infertility, the sperm may have to undergo special processing such as washing or concentration before exposure to the oocyte. When the oocyte is judged to be mature, it is mixed with the sperm for 18 hours. At the end of this time, the embryo is incubated for another 24 hours or so before being placed into the uterus.

4. **Embryo Transfer.** The conceptus is placed into the uterus at the two- to eight-cell stage. A tiny plastic tube with the embryo inside is placed through the cervix and then flushed out with fluid. This is an outpatient procedure that involves minimal discomfort. The woman is generally asked to lie flat on her back for 4 to 6 hours after the embryo is returned to the womb.

Just how effective is IVF? **PEARL: The pregnancy rate per cycle cited in a report from 281 fertility clinics in the United States was an overall 24% per cycle. Of these pregnancies, roughly 20% resulted in ectopic pregnancies or miscarriages and almost 30% were multiple births.** Most facilities actually put three or four embryos into the uterus in the hope that one will take hold and thrive.

Other variations of assisted reproductive technologies include gamete intrafallopian tube transfer (GIFT), in which sperm are placed near the fallopian tube during laparoscopy at the time of ovulation, and zygote intrafallopian tube transfer (ZIFT), in which the embryo is fertilized and placed into the fallopian tube rather than the uterus.

## ENDOMETRIOSIS

A neoplasm of the endometrial lining, endometriosis is unique among human diseases. **PEARL: Endometriosis combines a mixture of benign and malignant characteristics: the endometrial tissue retains its normal appearance and function but spreads beyond the organ in which it belongs. Endometriosis is almost never fatal, but it is the source of significant morbidity in terms of pain and infertility.**

*CONTROVERSY: There are at least four theories to explain the spread of endometrial cells beyond the uterine lining: lymphatic spread, hematogenous spread, retrograde menstruation, and metaplastic transformation of the peritoneal lining into endometrium.*

### Diagnosis

Endometriosis most commonly spreads to the pelvis but has been reported in the umbilicus, lung, intestines, cervix, and vagina. Within the pelvis, the usual site of endometriosis is in the cul-de-sac and along the uterosacral ligaments.

*CONTROVERSY: An elaborate staging system for this disease has been developed by the American Fertility Society, but in clinical practice, the disease stages correlate only poorly with patient complaints.*

There may be a weak familial tendency to develop endometriosis, but family history is not usually very helpful in deciding what to do for a particular patient.

*CONTROVERSY: Mild endometriosis that does not cause obvious scarring of the tubes or pelvis has been implicated in infertility, but the relationship, if any, is poorly understood.*

The classic history for endometriosis is the development of secondary dysmenorrhea, typically when the woman is in her late 20s or early 30s. Pain several days before the onset of menses is also particularly suspicious. Physical examination can suggest the presence of endometriosis but cannot establish the diagnosis. Suspicious findings include tenderness or nodularity on palpation of the uterosacral ligaments during the rectovaginal exam. On those rare occasions when endometriosis exists outside the peritoneal cavity, diagnosis depends on biopsy. Endometriosis is usually diagnosed at the time of laparoscopy that is performed to investigate pelvic pain or infertility. It is recognized by its characteristic "powder-burn" bluish lesions. The lesions are often so distinctive that many surgeons do not bother to biopsy them, although a pathology report may be useful for questionable abnormalities. Other manifestations of endometriosis that are visible at the time of laparoscopy include reddish growths on the peritoneal surfaces, scarring with adhesions around the pelvic organs, or holes in the peritoneal coverings.

## Treatment

The ultimate cure for endometriosis is the removal of the uterus and both ovaries, followed by hormone replacement therapy.

*CONTROVERSY: It is widely believed that exogenous hormones simply do not sustain endometriosis, as do normally functioning ovaries, although this theory has not been rigorously tested in the literature.*

Unfortunately this cure is not acceptable for many patients, typically women in their childbearing years. Medical and surgical alternatives often have limited success.

Oral contraceptive pills seem to suppress the spread of endometriosis, presumably because of their progestin-dominant effect on endometrium. In the same way that they suppress endometrial development within the uterus, they seem to do so throughout the body. In practice, these pills may inhibit the worsening of endometriosis, but they usually do not cause it to regress. Occasionally, continuous progestin treatment (orally, intramuscularly, or by implants) might be a more effective alternative, but rigorous comparisons of efficacy have not been performed.

Danazol, a weak androgen, has also been used to treat endometriosis, using doses varying from 100 mg to 800 mg daily for 6 to 9 months. The side effects of weight gain, decreased breast size, acne, hirsutism, hot flashes, and depression can be problematic.

Another class of drugs, the GnRH analogs leuprolide acetate (Lupron) and nafarelin acetate (Synarel), induce a menopausal state. Estrogen and progestin levels fall precipitously, and after several months, endometriosis lesions often seem to shrink or disappear. The problem is that when these drugs are stopped, the disease usually returns. As a result, GnRH analogs are typically used in conjunction with and before surgery. **PEARL: Endometriosis usually regresses permanently in the menopause, with or without HRT.**

The palliative surgical approach to endometriosis consists of physical destruction of the endometrial implants. Because these implants are often near or on vital structures, however, much judgment is required in deciding which lesions to ablate. In current practice, the lesions are destroyed with either laser or electrocautery via laparoscopy. Patients with substantial pain from endometriosis can also have selective destruction of nerves such as those that run near the uterosacral ligaments, or a pre-sacral neurectomy. These procedures usually provide only partial relief.

## Adenomyosis

Although it is not considered a variation of endometriosis, adenomyosis also involves endometrium growing where it is not naturally found—in this case, into the myometrium. A classic presentation would be a woman who presents with years of very heavy menses and severe dysmenorrhea, and who has a slightly enlarged, boggy uterus on exam. The diagnosis can be confirmed only at time of hysterectomy, although a deep biopsy taken during hysteroscopy can sometimes suggest it. Medical management of patients with suspected adenomyosis typically involves suppression of ovulation by oral contraceptive pills.

# 11
## CHAPTER

# *The Gynecologic Oncology Clinic*

Generally speaking, gynecologists deal with neoplasms of seven organs: the vulva, vagina, cervix, uterus, ovaries, placenta, and occasionally, the breasts. The vagina is one of the most uncommon sites of primary malignancy in the body. Treatment of vaginal neoplasms is similar to treatment of either cervical or vulvar cancer, depending on the site of the lesion. Fallopian tube cancer is similarly very rare. When it occurs, it is usually an adenocarcinoma and is typically treated similarly to ovarian cancer.

## VULVAR NEOPLASMS

**PEARL: Most vulvar lesions are benign, although the diagnosis usually can be established only by skin biopsies.** The two most common premalignant lesions are condyloma and its sequelae and lichen sclerosis. The three skin cancers—basal cell, squamous cell, and melanoma—can all occur on the perineum but rarely do so.

Condylomata can appear as warty, pediculated lesions or as flat, raised areas. Such human papillomavirus infections have been linked to premalignant changes of the vulvar skin known as vulvar intraepithelial neoplasia (VIN), which may be classified as mild, moderate, or severe.

**CONTROVERSY: Caution should be used in comparing the biology of VIN lesions to the corresponding grades in the cervix (see Chapter 8).**

In general, VIN is treated with local excision and 5-mm margins. The skin edges are simply reapproximated with absorbable sutures, usually leaving minimal scarring. Alternatively, the lesions can be destroyed with laser.

Two other specific premalignant diseases are occasionally encountered. Bowenoid papulosis is a specific variety of VIN III that appears as multiple red, brown, or purple papules. Another entity, Paget's disease, consists of white, flat lesions with sharp borders. Large, pale Paget cells on microscopic examination confirm the diagnosis. Paget's disease requires wide local excision with frozen section of the margins to be sure they are clear. In up to 20% of patients, the disease is associated with an adjacent adenocarcinoma; when present, these lesions require the same treatment as other invasive vulvar cancers.

Vulvar cancer is relatively rare; it causes 300 deaths among women each year in the United States. **PEARL: The staging criteria for vulvar cancer are contained in Appendix B and use the TNM classification based on surgical pathology.** Treatment for stage I vulvar cancer consists of radical vulvectomy with ipsilateral inguinal lymph node dissection. For stages II and III, radiation treatment or preoperative chemotherapy to shrink the tumor before surgery is often added to the foregoing treatment. Stage IV, widely metastatic disease, is typically associated with a poor prognosis and is managed with a variety of chemotherapy protocols.

The main method of diagnosing vulvar lesions remains the skin biopsy. Many of these vulvar abnormalities are multifocal and require several biopsies from different sites. After swabbing the area of interest with iodine, make a small skin wheal with local anesthetic. Then you may take a 3- to 5-mm punch biopsy. Alternatively, tent up the area using a forceps with teeth, and shave off a small portion of skin with a knife. Bleeding that does not stop with silver nitrate cautery may be controlled by one or two absorbable sutures.

# CERVICAL CANCER

Once neoplastic epithelium has penetrated below the basement membrane, the process is no longer a premalignant condition but rather invasive cancer. Beyond the history and physical, a chest x-ray study and CT scan of the pelvis and abdomen with intravenous contrast are used to help stage the cancer. Cystoscopy and bowel evaluation with sigmoidoscopy are prudent for those with stage II cancer and higher. **PEARL: Staging is a clinical assessment and is not changed by subsequent surgical pathology.**

In considering treatment for squamous cell cancers of the cervix, a condition referred to as microinvasive cancer requires special consideration. The most recent International Federation of Gynecology and Obstetrics (FIGO) definition from 1994 defines this entity as having a maximum depth of 5 mm and a maximum width of 7 mm. There is a growing consensus that those with depth of invasion of 3 mm or less can be treated with either cone biopsy or simple hysterectomy.

*CONTROVERSY: Those with invasion of 3 to 5 mm may also be able to be treated conservatively, but this approach is more controversial, with fewer data to support it.*

To treat more invasive cancers, a general rule of thumb is that patients with a stage of IIB (parametrial involvement) or higher are treated with radiotherapy.

*CONTROVERSY: Stage I and early stage II cancers may be treated either with radiation or with a radical hysterectomy in which the tissues adjacent to the cervix as well as the top fourth of the vagina are removed. Because the cure rates between radiotherapy and radical surgery are comparable, surgery is generally reserved for younger women in otherwise good health who desire preservation of ovarian function and, in some cases, better vaginal function.*

# UTERINE NEOPLASMS

The uterus has two types of tissue: the endometrium, which cycles each month, and the myometrium, the smooth muscle wall of the uterus. Both are subject to the development of benign and malignant tumors.

## Endometrial Neoplasms

Benign tumors of the endometrium are known as endometrial polyps. These polyps typically cause mid-cycle spotting or menorrhagia, but they are not common. They can be diagnosed occasionally during pelvic ultrasound exams but a more sensitive test is thought to be the hysterosonogram, in which water is injected into the uterine cavity while a vaginal ultrasound exam is being performed. The most sensitive procedure of all for diagnosing intrauterine lesions remains hysteroscopy. Endometrial polyps may be multiple but are not considered a premalignant lesion.

Endometrial cancer is newly diagnosed in 15,000 women each year in the United States and causes approximately 3000 deaths annually. Typically considered a slow-growing malignancy, many, although perhaps not all, endometrial cancers pass through discrete premalignant stages.

The three common hyperplasias, or pathologic thickenings, of the endometrium are cystic hyperplasia, adenomatous hyperplasia, and adenomatous hyperplasia with atypia. Cystic hyperplasia is not thought to be premalignant. Adenomatous hyperplasia may be an early premalignant lesion, although it usually is easily reversed by cyclic progestins. These medications include monthly injections of Depo-Provera or 20 mg daily of Provera (medroxyprogesterone acetate) for 3 to 6 months. An alternative is Megace (megestrol acetate) 40 mg orally, two to four times daily. Once diagnosed, follow-up endometrial biopsies should be obtained at 3- to 6-month intervals to ensure regression of the abnormality. Adenomatous hyperplasia with atypia is believed to be a more serious lesion; perhaps 25% of women with this condition will subsequently develop invasive cancer.

*CONTROVERSY: Medical treatment of women who have adenomatous hyperplasia with atypia is more controversial. In some cases, hysterectomy may be appropriate. Patients with this type of lesion diagnosed at the time of an office biopsy might benefit from a hysteroscopy and fractional D&C, because some may have a coexisting endometrial cancer.*

**PEARL: In considering treatment recommendations for women with atypia, age should be a factor because it is thought that women near the menopause or beyond may be at higher risk for developing invasive cancer than younger women with a similar lesion.**

Endometrial cancer usually causes irregular or abnormal bleeding. Its incidence peaks in the sixth decade of life, and most patients present with stage I (see Appendix B). Staging is based on surgical pathology. Prognosis and treatment recommendations are based on differentiation of the tumor, which, in turn, corresponds to invasiveness.

*CONTROVERSY: In general, women with anything more abnormal than well-differentiated, minimally invasive cancer benefit from pelvic and periaortic lymph node biopsies to assess the spread of disease. Those with positive nodes typically receive external radiation treatment. Whether the nodes are positive or not, it is common practice to offer women with cancer invading the myometrium intravaginal radiation treatment a few weeks after surgery. This treatment seems to reduce the most common sort of recurrence at the top of the vaginal cuff.*

## Myometrial Neoplasms

A benign tumor of the uterine wall is known as a fibroid tumor, or leiomyoma. Fibroids can cause a variety of symptoms depending on their size and location. Submucous myomas commonly present as a cause of heavy periods or frequent bleeding. Intramural or subserous fibroids can cause pressure on adjacent organs, although this is not usually an issue until their size becomes extreme. Degenerating fibroids that have outgrown their blood supply can cause pain, a problem most commonly seen during pregnancy. Some estimates suggest that 50% of women have fibroids. Rarely, they can be a cause of infertility or miscarriage, but this is typically a diagnosis of exclusion.

**PEARL: Fibroids are not premalignant lesions and do not warrant treatment unless they cause symptoms.** Most women with a leiomyoma do not need any treatment.

**CONTROVERSY: In the past, some authors suggested that a hysterectomy should be recommended for a uterus that has reached the size of a 12-week pregnancy, or for "rapidly growing fibroids," but in general, these doctrines are no longer valid.**

In symptomatic women, treatment generally consists of surgery. The GnRH agonists can cause fibroids to shrink by up to 30%, but they often regrow after suppressive therapy has stopped. A more common practice is to use medical management to facilitate a myomectomy (removal of individual tumors) or a vaginal hysterectomy. Depending on the size and location of the fibroids, a myomectomy can be perfomred via laparoscopy, hysteroscopy, or laparotomy. When offering a patient myomectomy, it is worth remembering the patient's original complaint (e.g., abnormal or heavy bleeding). **PEARL: Simply removing the fibroids may not resolve the patient's symptoms completely.** Of course, a hysterectomy is sure to cure any complaints remotely related to leiomyoma.

## Sarcomas

By definition, the malignancies of the myometrium are sarcomas. Fortunately, they are rare. The most common sarcoma almost always has widely metastasized by the time of diagnosis. Removal of the uterus is the basis of any curative treatment, which usually also includes chemotherapy for disease outside the uterus.

Uterine sarcomas can arise from the endometrium, myometrium, or supporting and connective tissues. **PEARL: Homologous tumors contain tissues normally present in the uterus, whereas heterologous tumors have components foreign to the uterus.** The mixed mesodermal sarcoma is the most common type among the sarcomas. Treatment for all sarcomas generally consists of hysterectomy with removal of both ovaries. Because radiation therapy has not been shown to improve survival, current efforts focus on chemotherapy protocols, but no regimen has yet proven to be of great value.

# OVARIAN NEOPLASMS

There are dozens of types of ovarian tumors. Only the more common ones are described here. These tumors are traditionally divided according to the three different tissues of origin within the ovary: epithelial cells, stromal cells, and germ cells.

## Epithelial Cell Tumors

Ovarian epithelial cells occupy the capsule of the ovary and provide the architectural support for the oocytes and the stromal cells that surround them. **PEARL: Tumors arising in epithelium may account for up to 70% of all ovarian neoplasms.** The benign tumors are serous and mucinous cystadenomas and Brenner tumors. Mucinous cystadenomas occasionally grow very large. Brenner tumors, also known as transitional cell tumors, are usually solid. All three tumors also have malignant varieties.

## Stromal Cell Tumors

Stromal cells constitute the hormonally active tissue of the ovary. The few ovarian tumors that secrete hormones are typically derived from these cells. Examples include granulosa cell tumors and thecomas, which can produce estrogen, and Sertoli-Leydig cell tumors, which can produce androgens.

## Germ Cell Tumors

The mature, benign variety of germ cell tumor is also called a dermoid cyst or a cystic teratoma. Cartilage, hair, and teeth can form in these tumors. A subtype of this tumor is known as struma ovarii; these rare tumors consist of thyroid tissue and can, in a small minority of cases, produce enough thyroid hormone to cause thyrotoxicosis. A variety of malignancies can arise from germ cells, including:

- **Dysgerminoma.** Uniquely sensitive to radiation

therapy and chemotherapy, this is one of the few ovarian malignancies in which removal of both ovaries may not always be necessary.

- **Endodermal sinus tumor (yolk sac tumor).** An aggressive malignancy, alpha-fetoprotein has proven to be a useful tumor marker.
- **Immature cystic teratoma.** As with its benign counterpart, the tumor has a variety of histologic entities. Its malignant behavior is related to the amount of mitotic activity and degree of differentiation.
- **Gonadoblastoma.** This tumor typically occurs in a congenitally abnormal gonad, such as in patients with gonadal dysgenesis, and may exist concomitantly with other germ cell tumors.

## Diagnosis

The most common ovarian malignancy involves epithelial cells. The incidence increases rapidly after age 45, peaking at age 75 to 79. **PEARL: Ovarian cancer is staged through surgery, and most cases are first diagnosed in stage III, when they have already metastasized.** A genetic predisposition to ovarian cancer has been identified in only a small percentage of individuals developing these malignancies. A single first-degree relative with ovarian cancer increases a woman's risk by only 5%.

A persistently enlarged ovary of 5–6 cm or more generally deserves investigation. Typically the patient should be advised to have a sonogram and return in 4 weeks for a repeat evaluation. If the physical findings are confirmed by ultrasound exam and there is no regression of the mass over 4 weeks, some type of surgical investigation such as laparoscopy is probably warranted. Of course, if the patient is having significant symptoms such as pain, if both ovaries appear enlarged, or if ascites is present, a delay of 4 weeks may not be necessary. The role of CA-125, a tumor marker commonly elevated in ovarian cancer, has yet to be established in screening for those without disease. Clearly, it is not an appropriate screening test in women without signs or symptoms of ovarian cancer, because it lacks both sensitivity and specificity.

*CONTROVERSY: The appropriateness of looking for CA-125 in evaluating patients with adnexal masses is not clear, but many gynecologists test for it anyway.*

The treatment of ovarian cancer consists of maximum surgical reduction of tumor mass, followed by radiation therapy for individuals with stage I or II disease and chemotherapy for those with stages III and IV.

A special case consists of "borderline tumor" or ovarian tumors with "low malignant potential." On microscopic examination, these tumors have greater epithelial proliferation than commonly seen in serous cystadenomas but no invasion is seen. **PEARL: As implied by its name, borderline tumor falls between purely benign and malignant.** Occasionally, normal ovaries can be preserved, particularly for those desiring future pregnancies.

## GESTATIONAL TROPHOBLASTIC DISEASE

Gestational trophoblastic disease is a rare placental tumor that has both benign and metastatic varieties. **PEARL: The benign form, hydatidiform mole, occurs in roughly 1 in 1500 pregnancies. Invasive moles occur 10 times less frequently, and choriocarcinoma occurs 1 in 40,000 times.** The classic symptoms of gestational trophoblastic disease are abnormal bleeding, uterine size much greater than dates, and hyperemesis gravidarum (excessive vomiting during pregnancy). The diagnosis is usually easily made by ultrasound exam: no fetus is identified and the placenta appears as grapelike clusters of tissue.

### Hydatidiform Mole

**PEARL: The benign variety of gestational trophoblastic disease, hydatidiform mole, does not metastasize.** Treatment consists of suction curettage with follow-up human chorionic gonadotropin (hCG) blood levels every 2 weeks until results are negative three consecutive times. **PEARL: A complete mole is thought to be 46,XX karyotype, with a 23,X being contributed by the fertilizing sperm,**

which subsequently doubles and replaces the oocyte's genetic material. Complete moles are never associated with a fetus. In contrast, partial moles usually have some fetal tissue and typically have a triploid karyotype, usually 69,XXY.

## Invasive Mole and Choriocarcinoma

Persistent disease is recognized either by the presence of obvious metastatic disease such as lesions visible in the vagina or on chest x-ray study, or by persistently elevated or rising hCG levels following treatment of hydatidiform mole. **PEARL: The distinction between invasive mole and choriocarcinoma is made at the time of pathologic examination of any biopsy specimens, but because these lesions notoriously bleed if they are disturbed surgically, histologic evaluation is not always possible.**

Therefore, treatment of invasive disease is predicated on establishing whether the patient is considered to be high risk or low risk. In low-risk patients, hCG levels are less than 40,000 mIU/mL, symptoms have persisted for less than 4 months, no brain or liver metastases exist, no prior chemotherapy was administered, and the pregnancy event is not a term delivery. High-risk patients, of course, are the converse. Low-risk patients typically are treated with single-agent chemotherapy (methotrexate), and multiagent chemotherapy is used for those at high risk. Both groups generally respond well to treatment and experience cure.

## BREAST DISEASE

In the United States, approximately 175,000 women are diagnosed with breast cancer annually, and about 41,000 die from it. Estimates of the risk of breast cancer over a woman's lifetime vary between 9% and 11%.

## History and Physical Examination

Because the breast is a mixture of glandular and adipose tissue, lumpiness, thickening, and irregularities are almost universal findings. **PEARL: The important**

**thing in breast examination is distinguishing benign lumps and irregularities from malignancies.** In taking the history, it is important to establish how long the lump has been present and whether it shrinks and swells. In general, a lump that shrinks during part of the month and swells at other times is probably normal glandular tissue. If a patient has had a lump for only a few days or weeks, it may be appropriate to have her return in 4 weeks before doing a workup to determine if the nodule persists. Breast cancer occurs most frequently in the upper, outer quadrant of either breast (Fig. 11–1).

The vast majority of malignancies are found by women themselves. It is very helpful to ask the patient if she has found any lumps that concern her. During the

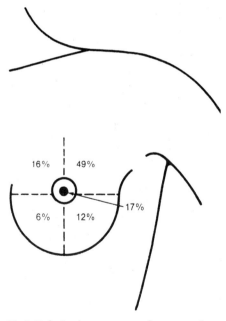

**Figure 11–1.** Relative breast cancer frequency, by quadrant (From DiSaia, PJ and Creasman, WT: Clinical Gynecological Oncology, ed. 4. Mosby–Year Book, St. Louis, 1993, p 474, with permission.)

physical exam, press the middle three fingers of your dominant hand gently against the breast tissue in a systematic fashion, moving circumferentially around the breast while stabilizing the area with the other hand. Take care to palpate the tail of the breast as it extends under the axilla. Note any localized tenderness, retraction, or breast discharge. In women aged 40 and older, it is helpful to perform the exam first with the woman sitting up and then lying down. While the patient is seated, having her clasp her hands behind her head is a useful technique to look for skin retraction. Breasts are commonly asymmetric, and this should not be confused with dimpling of the skin or its adherence to an underlying tumor, which is a relatively uncommon and late finding of breast cancer. While the patient has her hands behind her head, it is convenient to palpate the tail of the breast and axilla. You should also note any swollen lymph nodes.

## Breast Cancer Diagnosis

### *Mammography*

The American Cancer Society (ACS) recommends one mammogram for women between the ages of 35 and 40, a mammogram every 1 to 2 years from ages 40 to 50, and one annually thereafter. A mammogram is most useful as a screening test for unsuspected breast cancer. For a discrete, persistent lump (a so-called dominant mass), its utility is somewhat limited. **PEARL: A mammogram cannot prove that a dominant mass is not malignant.** This is not to say that a normal mammogram in a woman with a dominant breast mass has no predictive value at all. It can locate other suspicious lesions in either breast, and an *abnormal* mammogram can increase the suspicions that a specific lump is malignant, but for women who do have breast cancer, the mammogram will be abnormal only 80% of the time.

Women who have a first-degree relative with a history of premenopausal breast cancer probably should get more frequent screening, although this advice should be individualized. There is almost never a reason to perform a mammogram in a woman younger than 25 years of age; breast cancer in this age group is very uncommon, and a normal mammogram does not prove that a specific lump is benign.

### *Breast Aspiration*

Breast aspiration is a straightforward office procedure that can determine whether a dominant breast mass is solid or cystic. **PEARL: Because cystic masses are almost never associated with malignancy, in some circumstances, breast aspiration can be practically diagnostic.** Swab the skin over the lesion with an alcohol wipe, and then insert a syringe with a 21-gauge (or smaller) needle directly into the lump. Aspirate the lump. The diagnosis of breast cyst is made if fluid is obtained and the lump in question shrinks substantially. If this happens, the patient should be rechecked in 4 weeks to be sure that the nodule has not recurred. Whether the aspirated fluid should be sent for cytology is controversial; it usually provides little additional information. If it is to be sent, it can be spread thinly over a microscope slide and then fixed in the same way as a Papanicolaou (Pap) smear. The fluid can range from clear to yellow, green, or brown. Clear fluid in particular is reassuring, although discolored fluid also is often associated with benign lesions. In addition to the 4-week re-examination, the patient should be counseled to examine her breasts herself and to return for any new, persistent nodule.

### *Thin-Needle Aspiration Biopsy*

In thin-needle aspiration biopsy, which is a relatively new procedure, the examiner takes a specialized needle and syringe, and makes 10 to 20 rapid passes through the dominant mass while aspirating. In general, three or four separate efforts are made to help ensure that the suspicious area actually was sampled. Once again, normal histology cannot absolutely prove that a specific area is benign because one cannot be absolutely sure that the right area was sampled. In many situations, however, the procedure can be sufficiently reassuring that a breast biopsy can be deferred. The follow-up after thin-needle breast aspiration biopsy depends on the finding and clinical presentation.

## *Breast Biopsy*

Breast biopsy is generally considered the gold standard for diagnosing the malignancy status of a dominant mass. Local anesthesia is administered, the skin over the palpable lump is incised along the line of Langerhans (to minimize scarring), and the lump is removed. Often, frozen sections are obtained to give the patient a preliminary result, although in general, no further action is taken until the final pathology report is issued.

For suspicious areas that show up only on mammography, the radiologist generally performs needle localization, in which a thin wire or needle is placed in the breast to mark radiographically the area to be excised. After the tissue is removed, the tissue is then x-rayed again to be sure that it was the abnormality seen in the original mammogram.

## *Breast Self-Examination*

The ACS publishes a very detailed guide to breast self-examination. Unfortunately, with so much emphasis on technique, patients are easily discouraged. They often shrug their shoulders and state, "I do not know what I am feeling." It is helpful to emphasize that every breast has irregularities but that new lumps that persist for 4 weeks should be brought to the attention of a health professional.

## Genetics and Prevention

The ongoing revolution in biotechnology has brought forth two issues with regard to breast cancer. **PEARL: First, two genes (*BRCA1* and BRCA2) strongly linked to the development of breast and other gynecologic cancers have been discovered.** It has been estimated that women with either of these gene mutations have up to an 85% chance of developing breast cancer and an increased risk (perhaps not as high) of developing ovarian cancer.

*CONTROVERSY: Prophylactic mastectomies and oophorectomies are important options for patients with these genes, although our understanding of the role of these genes in the development of cancer remains limited.*

A second issue is the use of selective estrogen receptor modulators to prevent breast cancer in selected high-risk women. **PEARL: In a randomized trial involving over 13,000 women, tamoxifen reduced the rate of breast cancer development in high-risk women by 50% in comparison with placebo.** Tamoxifen attaches to some estrogen receptor sites and thereby reduces the effect of estrogen. Raloxifene is currently being evaluated for this role as well. The National Cancer Institute has distributed a risk assessment protocol (available on floppy disk) to assist clinicians in determining which women should be started on the prevention protocol. Risk factors involved in the formula include:

- History of breast abnormalities (ductal carcinoma in situ and locular carcinoma in situ)
- Age (increasing age increases risk)
- Age at menarche (younger than age 12 increases risk)
- Age at first live birth (first term pregnancy after 30 or no term deliveries increases risk)
- Race (white women are at greater risk than black women)
- Breast cancer among first-degree relatives
- History of breast biopsies, regardless of actual pathology.

*CONTROVERSY: It is believed that the clinical decision to proceed with a biopsy identifies women at increased risk, although the precise mechanism is unclear.*

## Treatment of Breast Cancer

Once a malignancy has been diagnosed by histology, the issue then becomes how to treat it. Lumpectomy with radiation therapy has largely replaced mastectomy in recent years.

### *Lumpectomy and Radiation Treatment*

**PEARL: Lumpectomy with radiation treatment (breast conservation) yields the same cure rate as mastectomy for stages I and II breast cancers (tumor 5 cm or less in diameter, no distant metastases).** The lumpectomy consists of widely excising the malignant tumor and performing an ipsilateral axillary lymph node dissection and biopsy. After a few weeks of healing, the breast is then treated with 4500 to 5000 cGy of radiation in doses of 180 to 200 cGy per session.

### Mastectomy

When evaluating the results of surgical intervention, new procedures are compared with the radical mastectomy as described by Halsted in 1894. This procedure involves wide en bloc resection of the breast containing the tumor together with the underlying pectoral muscles and the axillary lymph nodes. In addition to cosmetic concerns, this operation leaves 30% of patients with chronic arm edema. As a result, the modified radical mastectomy, which leaves the chest muscles intact, is often performed instead of the procedure as originally described.

*CONTROVERSY: Interestingly enough, radical mastectomy, modified radical mastectomy, and lumpectomy with radiation therapy all seem to yield the same cure rates.*

### Chemotherapy

In deciding whether to recommend chemotherapy, three factors are commonly considered: the presence or absence of estrogen receptors in the tumor, and the degree of spread (i.e., positive or negative lymph nodes).

**PEARL: There are two types of chemotherapy, hormonal and cytotoxic.** A common protocol for cytotoxic agents is the use of cyclophosphamide, methotrexate, and 5-fluorouracil in 6 to 12 monthly cycles. Tamoxifen, which attaches to estrogen receptor sites and reduces the effect of estrogen, is the agent most commonly used in hormonal therapy.

In general, premenopausal women with positive lymph nodes are often advised to undergo cytotoxic chemotherapy because premenopausal disease is particularly aggressive. Postmenopausal women with positive lymph nodes and a positive estrogen receptor assay are commonly treated with tamoxifen. Whether any group of women with negative nodes would benefit from chemotherapy, either cytotoxic or hormonal, is being studied. It should be noted that for women with distant disease (beyond the ipsilateral lymph nodes), treatment is regarded as primarily palliative.

# 3
### PART

# *The Operating Room*

# 12

# Surgical Instruments, Materials, and Techniques

The first visit to an operating room can be an overwhelming experience. This brief guide to commonly used instruments and materials should remove some of the unfamiliarity and help you to concentrate on what is happening rather than on how it is happening, which is less important.

## COMMONLY USED SURGICAL INSTRUMENTS, SUTURES, AND NEEDLES

**PEARL: Commonly used surgical instruments fall into three functional categories: cutting, retracting, and grasping.** Various types are described in Table 12–1.

Gynecologists typically use dissolving sutures in their surgeries, although nonabsorbable sutures are occasionally used. Suture gauge describes the diameter of the suture. Its nomenclature is somewhat confusing. Smaller gauge sutures are designated by a number followed by a dash and a zero. However, the zero is tradi-

## Table 12–1. SURGICAL INSTRUMENTS

| Instrument | Description |
|---|---|
| **Cutting Instruments: Knives** | |
| #10 blade | Large, curved; most commonly used |
| #11 blade | Pointed, triangular; for small, precise incisions |
| #15 blade | Small, curved |
| **Cutting Instruments: Scissors** | |
| Mayo | Curved, thick blades; cuts heavy tissue |
| Metzenbaum | Curved, thin blades; dissection; cuts thin tissue |
| Suture | Thick, straight blades; suture cutting dulls blades |
| **Retractors** | |
| Haney | Large, right-angle retractor; useful in vaginal hysterectomy |
| Deaver | Straight handle, curved blade; for abdominal wall |
| Malleable | Can be bent to conform to situation |
| Army-Navy | Right-angle blades on both ends |
| Richardson | Similar to Army-Navy retractor except that tips are slightly curved; used in opening and closing abdomen |
| **Grasping Instruments** | |
| Forceps | With and without teeth |
| Adson forceps | Small, delicate; with and without teeth |
| Hemostats | Straight and curved; for clamping blood vessels |
| Curved-6 | 6-inch curved clamp |
| Curved-8 | 8-inch curved clamp |
| Kocher clamp | Straight clamp with teeth at end |
| Heaney clamp | Heavy clamp with teeth near but not at tip; straight and curved; clamps large tissue bundles |
| Ring forceps | Long, straight; often used to hold sponges |
| Babcock clamp | Ends are half circles; grasps fallopian tubes |
| Allis clamp | Flared end with teeth; provides firm grasp |

tionally referred to as the letter "O." **PEARL: For small-gauge sutures, *in*creasing numbers indicate *de*creasing suture diameter.** For instance, 3–0 suture is smaller than 2–0 suture. To make matters more confusing, larger gauge sutures are designated by the word "number" before the numeral and these become larger in size with increasing number. For instance, #2 suture is *bigger* than #1 suture. (Both are huge and not commonly used in gynecologic surgery, however.)

Only a few types of absorbable sutures are commonly used in gynecology. Plain suture (untreated mammalian intestine) is the most rapidly absorbed and weakens significantly after a few days. Chromic suture consists of mammalian intestine strips specially treated with chromic salts. This type of suture maintains its strength somewhat longer—7 to 10 days. Vicryl and Dexon are polyglycolic acid suture (made by different companies). These sutures maintain 50% of their strength at 3 weeks and take 2 to 3 months to resorb totally. Examples of nonabsorbable sutures include silk, nylon, and Tevdek.

Needles are generally either straight or curved (Fig. 12–1). Two of the curved needles, ⅜ circle and ½ circle, are used frequently, whereas ¼ and ⅝ circle are used only in special circumstances. The shaft of the needle may be circular; this is called a taper-point needle and is used for sewing easily penetrated tissue such as peritoneum or bowel (Fig. 12–2). Other needles, called cutting needles, are triangular or polygonal in shape and typically have one of the angles sharpened to facilitate tissue penetration. The conventional cutting needle has a sharpened inside edge and is used for sewing fascia and skin. An atraumatic needle is one in which the suture is wedged into the shaft of the needle rather than being threaded through an eye at the end, as it is in sewing needles for clothes. Pop-off needles have suture affixed in such a way that sudden, moderate force applied to the needle will remove it from the suture.

## LAPAROSCOPIC INSTRUMENTS

Various unique instruments are used for laparoscopy. The first is the Veress needle, a long steel tube with a sharp tip that is covered by a spring-loaded

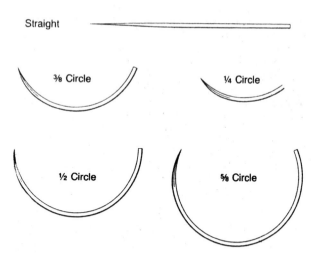

Straight

⅜ Circle

¼ Circle

½ Circle

⅝ Circle

**Figure 12–1.** Suture needles. (From Anderson, RM and Romfh, RF: Technique in the Use of Surgical Tools. Appleton-Century-Crofts, New York, 1980, p 198, with permission of the McGraw-Hill Companies.)

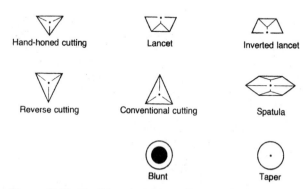

Hand-honed cutting

Lancet

Inverted lancet

Reverse cutting

Conventional cutting

Spatula

Blunt

Taper

**Figure 12–2.** Needle cross-sections. (From Anderson, RM and Romfh, RF: Technique in the Use of Surgical Tools. Appleton-Century-Crofts, New York, 1980, p 199, with permission of the McGraw-Hill Companies.)

sheath. In theory, the sharp tip is exposed only when it encounters significant resistance such as that offered by abdominal fascia. The same principle covers the much larger (5-mm to 12-mm) trocars that are used to guide the operating sheaths into the abdomen. Typically, these are introduced only after the abdomen has been sufficiently insufflated with carbon dioxide gas. The insufflators themselves usually have three gauges, which the surgeon monitors. The most important gauge measures abdominal pressure. Usually, it is desirable to keep this pressure below 20 mm Hg; higher pressures may mean that the sheath introducing carbon dioxide gas is not free in the abdomen but rather is in an enclosed space such as a hollow viscus or a mass of scar tissue. The other two gauges measure the volume of gas introduced and the flow rate.

In addition to the laparoscope itself, a variety of other instruments may be placed through the various size sheaths. These include Babcock clamps, staple applicators, scissors, and cautery devices. The most rapidly expanding part of the market is disposable instruments.

## LASERS AND
## ELECTROSURGICAL DEVICES

*CONTROVERSY: Lasers provide another method of cutting and cauterizing, but because they are expensive, technically temperamental, and cumbersome, they rarely offer significant advantages over alternative instruments. The advantage they do offer is chiefly depth control of tissue injury.*

In some sense, the laser was always a metaphoric hammer looking for a nail. Ironically, for abdominal and gynecologic surgery, technologic advances have largely relegated lasers to highly specialized, limited applications.

The carbon dioxide laser is typically used for destroying the transformation zone of the cervix and large condylomata of the lower genital tract. The carbon dioxide laser is invisible and thus requires a second, low-power helium-neon laser to provide a visible, red aiming point. The usefulness of the carbon dioxide laser is limited because it cannot penetrate blood.

The yttrium-aluminum-garnet (YAG) laser is capable of tissue destruction down to 4 mm, much deeper than the carbon dioxide laser. This is actually a disadvantage and has been circumvented through the use of sapphire tips that limit the depth of destruction. Unfortunately, the laser tips get hot and require constant cooling with a high-flow gas stream, typically nitrogen. This laser is sometimes used to destroy endometriosis because it is absorbed by darkly pigmented tissue and, with the sapphire tips, has a precisely controlled effect. The potassium-titanyl-phosphate (KTP) laser is similar to the YAG laser with respect to its precision.

It is important to know which type of laser is in use in the operating room. Laser light is easily reflected, and different wavelengths require different types of eye protection.

Electrosurgical devices are much less expensive than lasers and are easier to maintain. For laparoscopic surgery, they have largely replaced lasers for both cutting and cautery. **PEARL: The most commonly used electrosurgical devices are unipolar and require a ground. The current travels from the tip of the cautery device to the ground.** With bipolar cautery, the current passes between the two tips of the cautery instrument. Bipolar cautery is occasionally used in tubal ligations and for controlling bleeding from small vessels.

The type of current generated by unipolar cautery devices varies, depending on the desired effect. When cutting is chiefly desired, continuous current is generated so that the water in cells adjacent to the tip heats very quickly, causing these cells to burst. This prevents conduction of heat into the deeper tissue. During cautery procedures, the current is generated in pulses, allowing time for the heat to be conducted away from the site.

When using electrosurgery, it is important to ground the patient properly so that the current leaves the patient in a controlled manner. The chief drawbacks of electrosurgery are limited control over the depth of tissue destruction and the ever-present possibility that the current will not flow in the expected path but rather will damage tissue adjacent to the field of surgery. The generators are now so well engineered, however, that the uncontrolled flow of current (a highly undesirable event) is extremely uncommon.

## SURGICAL TECHNIQUE

There are many books on surgical technique, so only a few words are in order here. The most important objective in learning surgery is to understand the goal of the operation and the individual steps used to reach that goal. **PEARL: Anticipating the next step is absolutely necessary for surgical proficiency.**

A scalpel should be held with the thumb opposing the other four fingers so that steady downward pressure can be maintained, particularly when incising the abdominal wall. Stabilize the tissue to be incised with the nondominant hand, and try to stay in the same vertical plane as the incision is made deeper into the tissue. Clamps with locking teeth should be fully closed. When cutting suture, it is desirable to stabilize the dominant hand with the other (if possible) and simply use the tips of the scissors. Never cut what you cannot see.

The suture material being tied determines the specific type of knot to be used. For instance, sutures that hold knots well, such as plain and chromic catgut, can be secured with three half-hitches. Suture material prone to slippage, such as Vicryl, Dexon, and polydioxanone (PDS), are often better secured with a surgeon's knot (two initial throws) followed by three or four additional half-hitches. Leave substantial suture material beyond the knot when cutting excess suture, particularly in deeper layers, where the excess will not protrude through the skin.

# 13
## CHAPTER

# *Specific Operations*

Five commonly performed operations are described here. These descriptions are but one way to do these operations. Seldom does any operation conform entirely to the printed word in a textbook. One special tip for students: the lump near (or in) the bladder during abdominal cases is the bulb of the Foley catheter. Actual dictation examples for these surgeries are contained in Appendix C.

## ABDOMINAL HYSTERECTOMY AND BILATERAL SALPINGO-OOPHORECTOMY

**PEARL: This procedure has three stages: entering the abdomen, removing the uterus, and closing the abdomen.**
Gynecologists make three common types of incisions: the vertical midline incision and two types of horizontal incisions, Pfannenstiel's incision and the Maylard incision. The vertical incision is made in the midline, typically from just above the symphysis pubis to just below the umbilicus. If needed, the incision can be extended by going around the umbilicus and then continuing upward. The layer after the skin, the fascia, is recognizable by its smooth, shiny, white surface. **PEARL: Occasionally, a weak and tenuous fascia, called Scarpa's fascia, appears within the adipose tissue. Do not confuse this type with the substantial rectus fascia beneath.**

Immediately underneath lie the rectus muscles, which can be bluntly separated from each other in the midline. Some patients also have a pyramidalis muscle on either side, sitting on top of the rectus muscles in the bottom half of the abdomen. Underneath the muscle layer lies the peritoneum. Approximately midway between the symphysis and the umbilicus lies the arcuate line, which delineates the bottom edge of the so-called posterior sheath (a portion of fascia enveloping the upper portion of the rectus muscles).

Both types of horizontal incisions are generally made 2 or 3 cm above the superior aspect of the symphysis pubis. **PEARL: With Pfannenstiel's incision, the abdominal muscles are dissected off the fascia above and below the transverse fascial incision. This permits separation of the muscles vertically in the midline. With the Maylard incision, the medial two thirds of the rectus muscles are incised bilaterally to permit access to the abdominal cavity.**

*CONTROVERSY: Recuperation from the Pfannenstiel and Maylard incisions is largely the same; the choice of transverse incision is usually made at the time of surgery, based on which appears easiest.*

Before the peritoneal cavity is entered, the preperitoneal fat is pushed away. Typically, the thin peritoneal tissues are grasped on either side of the midline with tissue forceps with teeth, and then they are gently incised with a knife. Care is taken that bowel is not immediately on the peritoneum, and the incision is made high enough in the abdomen to avoid the bladder, which sits at the bottom of the peritoneal lining as it turns away from the anterior abdominal wall to cover the visceral organs.

Once the incision is complete, the pelvis and abdomen are explored, and the abdominal wall is retracted (usually with a self-retaining retractor). The bowel is then packed away.

At this point, the uterus is grasped across either cornua by a clamp such as an 8-inch Kocher clamp. This technique provides for manipulation of the uterus as well as hemostasis for the proximal aspect of the fallopian tube, the ovarian suspensory ligament, and the round ligament. The round ligament is clamped distally with a 6-inch Kocher and then the ligament is cut with a Mayo scissors and ligated distally with #0 Vicryl (Fig. 13–1*A*). The suture is held long with a straight hemostat for later identification. The peritoneum is then cut with a Metzenbaum scissors toward the dome of the bladder, taking care to avoid the underlying uterine vessels and the bladder itself (Fig. 13–1*B*). The incision is also extended upward to permit visualization of the infundibulopelvic ligament and its blood vessels. **PEARL: With the retroperitoneal space opened in this fashion, the ureter can be palpated or visualized, or both, deep in the pelvis on the medial leaf of the broad ligament.** A hole is then made in the medial peritoneum underneath the in-

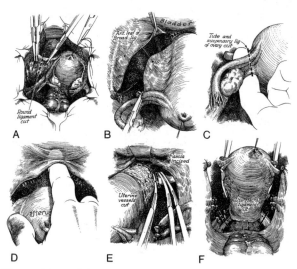

**Figure 13–1.** Abdominal hysterectomy. **A,** Clamping and dividing the round ligament. **B,** Dividing the vesico-uterine peritoneum. **C,** Site of division of the fallopian tube and ovarian suspensory ligament (with ovarian preservation). **D,** Dissection of the bladder off the lower uterine segment. **E,** Clamping and dividing uterine blood vessels. **F,** Uterine vessels and cardinal ligament cut and ligated. Location of uterosacral ligaments (from posterior aspect of uterus). (Modified from Wheeless, CR Jr: Atlas of Pelvic Surgery Copyright © Lea & Febiger, Philadelphia, 1981, pp 213 and 215, with permission. Illustrations by John Parker.)

fundibulopelvic ligament. The blood vessels here are then doubly clamped, typically with a curved Heaney clamp proximally and a curved-6 clamp just distal to the first clamp. The tissue is then cut between the two clamps, usually with Mayo scissors. The pedicle is secured by a pulley suture of #0 Vicryl (both strands of the suture are wrapped around the front of the pedicle and tied in back as the Heaney clamp is removed). A free tie of #0 Vicryl is then placed just distal to the first tie (the pulley suture). This double ligation of the infundibulopelvic ligament is a safeguard against postoperative bleeding should one of the sutures become loose. The curved-6 clamp is left on the distal pedicle, which is a portion of the surgical specimen. The process is repeated on the other side. If ovarian preservation is desired, the ovarian suspensory ligament and fallopian tube are double clamped, divided, and suture ligated close to the uterine cornua (Fig. 13–1C).

Once the upper attachments of the uterus are freed, the bladder is bluntly and sharply dissected off the uterus and retracted (Fig. 13–1D). Peritoneal tissue covering the uterine arteries is cut away anteriorly and posteriorly, a process also known as "skeletonizing the vessels." The uterine artery is then double clamped with a curved Heaney clamp distally and a curved-6 clamp proximally (Fig. 13–1E). Some surgeons actually place three clamps on these large vessels. Alternatively, some surgeons place only a single clamp on both sides before dividing them. The vessels are then divided with a Mayo scissors placed at the edge of the pedicle, brought around the clamp, and then placed again through the middle of the pedicle (a fixation suture or Haney suture).

**CONTROVERSY: Some surgeons doubly ligate the uterine artery, although many do not because of the relatively confined space.**

Additional branches of the uterine vessels are then double clamped, divided, and suture ligated distally on either side. At this point, the cardinal ligament, which attaches laterally to the upper portion of the cervix, is clamped, divided, and suture ligated. The uterosacral ligament, which attaches to the lower uterine segment posteriorly, is clamped, separated on either side, cut, and suture ligated (Fig. 13–1*F*). These sutures are typically held long for subsequent identification.

The uterus can now be removed from the patient by clamping across both lateral vaginal apices with curved Heaney clamps and cutting the cervix away from the vagina. The vaginal cuff can then be sewn closed with either a running locking suture of #0 Vicryl or a series of interrupted figure-of-eight sutures of #0 Vicryl. Some surgeons actually leave the vaginal cuff open so that fluids can drain out of the abdomen more easily. Hemostasis in this case is accomplished by placing a running, locking suture circumferentially over the rough edge of the vagina. (The cuff closes on its own in a few days.)

**CONTROVERSY: In closing the abdomen, surgeons may reapproximate both layers of peritoneum, one layer, or neither. Several studies have found no benefit to closing the peritoneum specifically as a separate layer. If it is closed, a smaller gauge suture such as 3–0 Vicryl is used.**

Before closing, each of the pedicles is inspected for hemostasis and the pelvis is often irrigated. The fascia is then closed with two separate running sutures of #0 Vicryl after checking the underlying muscles for hemostasis.

**CONTROVERSY: Some gynecologists specifically close the subcutaneous tissue (typically with 3–0 plain suture), but this practice is gradually falling out of favor because some data have linked it to an increased risk of wound infections.**

Finally, the skin can be closed with staples or with a subcuticular suture (e.g., 4–0 Vicryl).

# VAGINAL HYSTERECTOMY

A vaginal hysterectomy may be appropriate for women with a uterus the size of a 12-week pregnancy or less (a small grapefruit). With the patient prepped and draped in the dorsal lithotomy position, a pelvic exam under anesthesia is performed to confirm the size and position of the uterus. A weighted speculum is then placed into the vagina to hold the posterior wall out of the way while an assistant positions a right-angle retractor to keep the anterior wall out of the surgical field. At this point, a tenaculum is placed on the cervix to provide countertraction while a circumferential incision is made around the cervix close to the level of the internal os, just distal to the beginning of vaginal mucosa (Fig. 13–2*A*). With a combination of blunt dissection with a moist sponge and sharp dissection with a Metzenbaum scissors, the anterior cul-de-sac and then the posterior cul-de-sac are entered (Figs. 13–2*B*, *C*). The anterior cul-de-sac can be particularly troublesome because the bladder is in close proximity and the correct surgical plane between the uterus and bladder can be difficult to identify. It is desirable to enter

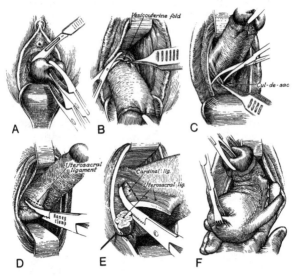

**Figure 13–2.** Vaginal hysterectomy. **A,** Incising the cervix. **B,** Incising the anterior cul-de-sac (vesico-uterine peritoneum). **C,** Incising the posterior cul-de-sac. **D,** Clamping and dividing the uterosacral ligament. **E,** Clamping and dividing the cardinal ligament. **F,** Inverting the uterus for better exposure of the round ligaments and fallopian tubes. (Modified from Wheeless, CR Jr: Atlas of Pelvic Surgery Copyright © Lea & Febiger, Philadelphia, 1981, pp 203 and 205, with permission. Illustrations by John Parker.)

both spaces early in the operation because this approach facilitates clamping of the subsequent pedicles and tends to reduce blood loss and operating time.

**PEARL: The middle portion of a vaginal hysterectomy consists of sequentially clamping and suture ligating the uterosacral ligament, the cardinal ligament, and the uterine blood vessels on both sides of the uterus (Figs. 13–2D, E).** This is opposite to the order in which these structures are secured during the abdominal hysterectomy. At some point, the surgeon will typically grasp the posterior aspect of the fundus and actually pivot the body of the uterus out of the vagina (Fig. 13–2F), making access to the upper uterine attachments easier. At the top of the uterus, the round ligament, fallopian tube, and ovarian suspensory ligament are often double clamped and double ligated much as the infundibulopelvic ligament is secured, as described for the abdominal hysterectomy. The uterus is then free from the patient. It is also possible to remove both ovaries simply by bringing them into the surgical field and then clamping the infundibulopelvic ligament. This procedure can be technically difficult, however, so that many surgeons do not guarantee a salpingo-oophorectomy to their patients at the time of vaginal hysterectomy.

With the uterus removed, some surgeons attempt to close the peritoneum with a circular running suture (e.g., 2–0 Vicryl). As with an abdominal hysterectomy, the vaginal cuff can be sewn closed or left open, depending on the preference of the surgeon. **PEARL: Vaginal hysterectomies are more prone to surgical site infections than abdominal hysterectomies.** For this reason, prophylactic antibiotics are often administered just before surgery (e.g., 1 g Ancef intravenous [IV] piggyback). An uncomplicated vaginal hysterectomy offers much faster recovery, however, because the abdominal musculature is not incised and the only suture line is perhaps 2 inches long in an area without muscles used for movement.

## LAPAROSCOPY

Laparoscopy can be used for either diagnosis or treatment. The most common setup for laparoscopy is the placement of the laparoscope through a 10-mm sheath placed just below the umbilicus, with the addition of a 5-mm sheath in the midline at the level of the pubic hair line, through which other instruments such as probes can be placed. For significant operative interventions, one or two 12-mm sheaths are placed into the abdomen lateral to either rectus muscle (and the inferior epigastric artery), an inch or so below the umbilicus.

At the outset of a laparoscopic procedure, the bladder is emptied with a catheter, and a pelvic exam is performed with the patient under anesthesia. The cervix is then exposed and grasped on the anterior lip with a single-tooth tenaculum, and a Rubin cannula is inserted (Fig. 13–3). A Rubin cannula is a hollow metal probe designed to be inserted into the cervical canal so that the uterus can be manipulated. An alternative is a plastic device with a deflated balloon at the end, known as a HUMI uterine manipulator. The balloon is inflated after the device has been inserted through the cervical canal, to aid in holding it in place. **PEARL: Perhaps the least traumatic way of manipulating the uterus is simply to place a ring forceps grasping a 4-by-4–inch sponge into the vagina so that the uterus can be pushed out of the way as needed.** This approach eliminates

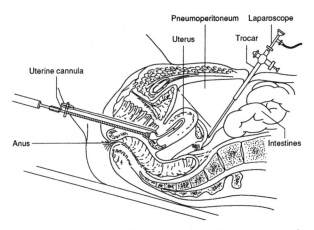

**Figure 13–3.** Gynecologic laparoscopy. (From Cavanaugh BM: Nurse's Manual of Laboratory and Diagnostic Tests, ed 3 Philadelphia, FA Davis, 1999, p 571, with permission.)

the risk of uterine perforation on insertion and vaginal bleeding when the instrument is removed.

After the uterine manipulator is secured, a Veress needle is placed through a small incision made immediately below the umbilicus. A syringe half filled with normal saline is used to aspirate to be sure the needle is not in a gas- or blood-filled place. The saline is then placed into the end of the Veress needle, and the abdomen is tented, creating negative pressure that should suction the drop into the needle if the needle tip is in the proper place.

**CONTROVERSY:** *Not all surgeons follow these steps, and surgical misadventures such as bowel or bladder perforation can occur (and will on occasion) no matter what precautions are taken.*

When the surgeon is satisfied with the needle placement, the abdomen is insufflated with 3 to 4 liters of carbon dioxide gas. After sufficient distension, the incision is enlarged transversely, and the Veress needle is removed. The 10-mm sleeve with trocar in place is then inserted into the abdomen. The trocar is removed and the laparoscope is inserted promptly to be sure that it is correctly located within the peritoneal cavity and that there is no obvious bleeding or injury. A second incision is made transversely in the midline at the level of the pubic hairline, through which a second sleeve with a trocar in place is inserted. **PEARL: With this second puncture, however, the tip of the trocar is observed directly through the laparoscope.** When properly positioned, the trocar is removed and the probe or other instrument is inserted.

At the end of the procedure, the probe is removed while being watched through the laparoscope and then the laparoscope itself is removed. The gas is allowed to escape through both sleeves, which are then also taken out of the incision. The method used to close these small wounds varies, but a typical technique is to place two simple interrupted sutures of 3–0 plain in the umbilicus and a single interrupted suture in the lower site.

**CONTROVERSY:** *For fascial incisions 11 mm or more in length, many surgeons will reapproximate the fascia with a suture such as #0 Vicryl to reduce the risk of an incisional hernia.*

When removing the vaginal instruments, care is taken to avoid excessive bleeding from the tenaculum site on the cervix. If bleeding is heavy, it responds readily to chemical cautery with application of silver nitrate.

Although it is an outpatient procedure, laparoscopy does have a small but serious complication rate. Bowel injuries and bleeding from vessel lacerations can and do occur.

*CONTROVERSY: A technique known as open laparoscopy, in which the fascia is entered under direct vision in the traditional fashion, has been advocated by some as a way to reduce complications, particularly in patients with prior surgery and a risk of adhesions. Little objective evidence supports the use of this approach, however, and there is no consensus on its utility.*

## DILATION, CURETTAGE, AND HYSTEROSCOPY

Often called a "DNC" by patients who are not really sure what is done during the procedure, dilation and curettage (D&C) should always include an examination of the uterine cavity with a hysteroscope.

*CONTROVERSY: Many view the hysteroscopy as often the most valuable aspect of the procedure for the patient who needs a D&C.*

With the patient in the dorsal lithotomy position, a pelvic exam is performed with the patient under anesthesia to confirm the orientation and size of the uterus. The cervix is then exposed and grasped on the anterior lip with a single-tooth tenaculum. A kevorkian curette is used to scrape the endocervical canal and obtain a specimen. Most of the sample remains behind in the mucus at the cervical os. This material can be collected readily by using an empty ring forceps to grasp this mucus and place it on a small piece of Telfa, which then goes to the pathology lab immersed in formaldehyde.

At this point, the uterus is sounded (measured) and

the cervix is dilated sequentially to 9 mm. A normal-size uterus typically measures less than 8 cm along its internal longitudinal axis. The hysteroscope (typically 8 mm in diameter with its sleeve) is inserted into the uterus, and copious irrigation fluid (preferably glycine) is used. Air bubbles and debris can be removed through a small polyethylene catheter inserted into one of the ports on the hysteroscope sheath. A small biopsy forceps can be inserted into this port to sample tissue of interest under direct vision.

After the hysteroscopy has been completed, sharp curettage is done by gently scraping all four sides of the uterus with the curette. **PEARL: Care must be taken not to push the curette forward with any force, as the uterus can easily be perforated.** Any tissue obtained is sent to the pathology lab separate from the endocervical curettage. At the end of the procedure, all the instruments are removed and the cervix is inspected for bleeding.

## BURCH PROCEDURE

Also known as a retropubic urethral suspension and similar in many ways to the Marshall-Marchetti-Krantz operation, the surgery begins with an abdominal incision that stops short of entering the peritoneal cavity. At this point, the space of Retzius, between the back of the symphysis pubis and the bladder, is entered. The fat overlying the vesicovaginal fascia and Cooper's ligament is then bluntly dissected away. It is often helpful to distend the bladder slightly with 100 to 200 mL of indigo carmine dye while at the same time clamping off the Foley drainage. At this point, the surgeon places his or her nondominant hand into the vagina to facilitate placing traction on the Foley as well as to push up on the periurethral tissue.

With the assistant providing exposure with sponge sticks (4-by-4-inch gauze folded in a ring forceps) and retractors, the surgeon places a suture into the vesicovaginal fascia 1 cm lateral to the proximal point of the urethra—the place where the urethra enters the bladder (demarcated by palpating the Foley bulb). **PEARL: This plane of the vesicovaginal fascia typically has a gray-**

white appearance and is relatively tough, particularly in comparison to the overlying adipose tissue commonly present.

*CONTROVERSY: Many surgeons place the suture through this tissue twice—a so-called "double throw." Both absorbable and nonabsorbable sutures have been used for this purpose, with each type having its advocates.*

A second suture is placed 1 cm lateral to the urethra, 1 cm distal to the first suture. The same procedure is then followed on the contralateral side so that the urethra is supported by two sutures on either side of it in the vesicovaginal fascia. The needle is left on the suture so that it can then be placed through Cooper's ligament, the tough, fibrous fascia inserting into the pubic symphysis. The distal urethral suture is placed through the medial aspect of Cooper's ligament while the proximal suture is placed 1 cm lateral to this. In this manner, the sutures do not cross or rub against each other. After this procedure has been done on both sides, the sutures are tied down in sequence by the assistant.

How much tension should be placed on these sutures? Unfortunately, there is no rigorously tested, reproducible answer. If too little tension is maintained, the patient's stress incontinence may not be helped. Excessive tightening, on the other hand, can result in prolonged urinary retention.

*CONTROVERSY: To test the tension, some physicians place a cotton swab in the urethra and then pull up on the sutures until the swab is parallel to the floor. Others leave a small amount of space between the urethra and the back of the symphysis.*

The fascia and skin can then be closed in the usual fashion. Some surgeons place a suprapubic catheter before closing the fascia. This can be done by filling the bladder with 400 mL of indigo carmine, making a stab wound a few centimeters away from the incision and then placing the catheter with trocar in place directly through the skin, fascia, and into the bladder. Most surgeons like to secure the catheter with a suture (such as 3–0 silk) in the skin.

**CONTROVERSY:** *An alternative to placing a suprapubic catheter at the time of a Burch procedure is teaching the patient before surgery to perform self-catheterization. A few physicians claim that they almost never have trouble with urinary retention after this procedure.*

Of course, the highly varying approaches and experiences with the operation underscore the difficulty of establishing long-term success rates from this procedure or any other anti-incontinence surgery.

# 14
## CHAPTER

# *Perioperative Issues*

Patients undergoing gynecologic surgery fortunately are usually in good health and do not need a great deal of special preparation. This chapter reviews only those preoperative and postoperative issues that are commonly encountered in gynecology.

## PREOPERATIVE CONSIDERATIONS

Women in good health who are younger than 50 years of age need only a complete blood count (CBC) in the way of preoperative testing. A urine pregnancy test within a few days of surgery is often a good idea as well and may be required in some hospitals. After age 50, many anesthesia departments also require a urinalysis, cardiogram, and liver function tests, along with electrolyte analysis. The guidelines vary among hospitals, but the trend is to order fewer lab tests routinely. Women with significant medical problems should get the appropriate preoperative consultation.

Patients should fast for at least 8 hours before surgery, although they can take critical medication orally with a sip of water. Women aged 40 and older undergoing inpatient surgery might benefit from some type of venous thrombosis prophylaxis. This generally comes in the form of thigh-high elastic thromboembolic disease (TED) hose, sequential compression boots, or heparin 5000 U subcutaneously every 12 hours. Heparin is generally reserved for those undergoing cancer surgery. Anyone in whom a vaginal incision into the peritoneal cavity is planned should also be given preoperative antibiotic prophylaxis (typically a low-cost cephalosporin such as Ancef, 1 or 2 g IV piggyback) and an iodine douche. Some surgeons also order preoperative enemas but this practice varies.

**PEARL: Although much gynecologic surgery is electively performed on healthy women, the American Society of Anethesiologists' physical status classification provides a good perspective because the categories have a strong association with surgical outcome (e.g., mortality):**

Class I: Healthy

ClassII: Mild disease. No functional limitations

Class III: Severe disease with limitations but not life-threatening

Class IV: Life-threatening disease

Class V: Death expected within 24 hours without surgery

The designation E is added onto the class to designate emergency surgery and is linked to a poorer outcome.

## SURGICAL CONSENT

Before surgery, surgical consent should be obtained from the patient. Ideally, this duty is the responsibility of the attending surgeon, but in a teaching environment, the surgeon may expect the house officer or, rarely, even a student to obtain this consent. The phrasing of this consent varies widely, even for the same operation. Also, although obtaining the consent ensures that the patient is provided with important information, in practice, this procedure does not seem to give patients the comfort that they may need. Aside from the fact that the decision to have surgery is a highly emotional, anxiety-charged issue, few patients have the scientific background to enable them to truly evaluate concepts of relative risk. It is often helpful to put the risks into perspective (i.e., they're usually uncommon) and also to review the benefits hoped for.

**PEARL: With these limitations in mind, patients should generally be counseled that "the risk of abdominal surgery includes but is not limited to the possibility of blood loss requiring blood transfusion, injury to abdominal organs requiring additional surgery to repair, and infection leading to other, more serious, complications."** Obviously, the degree of risk depends on the specific surgery being performed and specific complications can be emphasized or down-played as appropriate. For patients older than 40 years of age who undergo abdominal surgery, venous thrombosis is also at least a small possibility.

## POSTOPERATIVE ORDERS

Postoperative orders should address monitoring, eating, pain and nausea medication, and activities. For outpatients, typical orders would be:

1. Vitals per recovery room routine, then every 4 hours
2. IV 5% dextrose and lactated Ringer's (D5 LR) at 8-hour rate; discontinue when the patient tolerates oral liquids
3. Advance diet as tolerated
4. Pain medication
5. Nausea medication
6. Discharge when stable

The nurses usually have standing orders to notify the physician for fever, elevated pulse, or other untoward events. These notification orders can be written in but are not usually necessary if standing orders exist.

For inpatients having major abdominal surgery (e.g., hysterectomy), the immediate postoperative orders would be:

1. Vitals per recovery room routine, then every 4 hours
2. IV D5 LR at 8-hour rate
3. Nothing by mouth
4. Foley catheter to gravity drainage
5. Input and output every 8 hours
6. Getting up with assistance
7. Incentive spirometry every hour while awake
8. Thigh-high sequential compression boots

9. Hemoglobin/hematocrit in the morning
10. Physician to be notified for output less than 300 mL in 8 hours, pulse greater than 110 beats/min, or temperature greater than 101.0°F

*CONTROVERSY: A number of studies have shown no relationship between postoperative ileus and early feeding. Even so, many surgeons do not permit patients to be given a general diet until they have passed flatus.*

Twenty-four hours after surgery, most patients can have their Foley catheter removed and should be encouraged to ambulate in the halls with the help of a nurse. A general rule of thumb is that if a patient is eating and ambulatory, she can be discharged.

In today's managed care environment, each postoperative day needs to be justified by documenting the care that the patient is receiving that she could not provide for herself at home.

Patients with a suprapubic catheter who are undergoing postoperative bladder training require special orders:

1. Close the catheter when patient awakes. Leave the catheter open when the patient goes to sleep for the evening.
2. To check a residual, leave the catheter open for 5 minutes and then close it. Record what drained into the bag during those 5 minutes.
3. Record on flow sheet all voiding times, volumes, and residuals, together with the initials of the person making the measurements.
4. Patients may void as frequently as they like. If they have not voided or had a residual checked in 3 hours, they should attempt to void. Successful or not, a residual should be checked.

## POSTOPERATIVE PAIN RELIEF

Two common methods of inpatient pain relief are patient-controlled analgesia (PCA) and epidural narcotics. Although the orders for these modalities are often given by the anesthesiologist, it is helpful to know something about them. PCA consists of a computerized pump that can administer narcotics, typically morphine or Demerol, through IV push whenever the patient presses a button on a cable at the bedside. PCA permits frequent small dosing of narcotic and thus prevents large peaks and troughs. The result is that less medication is required than with intramuscular (IM) injections, and the patient experiences fewer side effects. The pump has a lockout mechanism that limits the maximum hourly dose that can be administered, to prevent overdoses.

Epidural narcotic administration also uses a computerized pump to provide a small, constant flow of narcotic (typically morphine or fentanyl) to the epidural space. This modality provides good pain relief with even lower doses of drug, so that side effects are limited.

Narcotics may still be ordered to be given by traditional IM administration. Roughly equivalent doses include morphine 10 mg, Dilaudid (hydromorphone) 1.5 mg, and Demerol (meperidine) 100 mg IM. These medications are typically given every 3 to 4 hours.

Once a patient is taking liquids orally, she can be given oral pain medication. Orally active narcotic agents, in decreasing order of potency, include Percocet (oxycodone and acetaminophen), Tylenol #3 (codeine and acetaminophen), and Darvocet-N 100 (propoxyphene napsylate and acetaminophen). The usual dosing is Percocet, 1 tablet every 4 hours; Tylenol #3, two tablets every 4 hours; and Darvocet-N 100, one tablet every 4 hours. An alternative to these narcotics is a potent antiprostaglandin, Toradol 10 mg, one tablet every 6 hours. Vicoprofen, a mixture of a narcotic with ibuprofen, is a particularly effective oral analgesic that can be prescribed without using a triplicate form.

The narcotics commonly cause nausea. Zofran (ondansetron hydrochloride), 4 mg IV push over 2 minutes preoperatively, has been associated with decreased postoperative nausea. Anzemet, 12.5 mg IV push every 6 hours, can also be used. Other antiemetics include prochlorperazine (Compazine), 10 mg IM every 6 hours; promethazine (Phenergan), 25 mg IM every 4 hours; and hydroxyzine (Vistaril), 50 to 75 mg every 4 hours.

## POSTOPERATIVE COMPLICATIONS

**PEARL: A postoperative fever is defined as a temperature of 100.4°F or greater measured twice, 6 hours apart.** Up to half of postoperative patients experience a fever in the first few days following surgery.

*CONTROVERSY: Although a substantial percentage of patients with postoperative fever do have an infection, many do not. For those without a microbial explanation for their fever, atelectasis (the collapse of the small airways) often has been ascribed as a cause, but the scientific evidence is scant.*

Many postoperative fevers have no known explanation, but the probability of an infection increases as the fever increases. Common sites of infection include the urinary tract, pneumonia, the skin incision, and an operative site such as the vaginal cuff.

Wound dehiscence, or breaking open of the surgical wound (i.e., the fascia), is more common in obese patients or those with chronic illnesses such as malignancy or diabetes. A specific suture technique, the Smead-Jones, has been linked to less risk of dehiscence. It involves placing the suture through the fascia and muscle in the far bites and into the anterior fascia in the near bites. Polyglycolic acid sutures, which take longer to be absorbed, are also associated with stronger wounds.

*CONTROVERSY: Debate continues over the relative strength of continuous sutures versus interrupted ones in the absence of evidence clearly supporting one technique over the other.*

**PEARL: A classic sign of wound dehiscence is the leaking of copious amounts of serosanguineous fluid from the incision.** When this occurs, the wound should be probed with a cotton swab to check for fascial defects. Small defects may be observed, but fascial gaps greater than 1 or 2 cm probably require reoperation.

One of the most serious complications following surgery is pulmonary embolism, which can still occur with some frequency despite prophylaxis. **PEARL: The**

**classic symptoms of an embolism include chest pain, dyspnea, tachypnea, and tachycardia, although many patients do not display them.** The key to diagnosis is a high degree of suspicion. Pulmonary angiography remains the gold standard for diagnosis, but a ventilation perfusion scan may be a useful screening tool that is less invasive.

*Appendixes*

# A

APPENDIX

# *World Health Organization Classification of Female Genital Mutilation**

| | |
|---|---|
| **Definition** | "Female genital mutilation comprises all procedures involving partial or total removal of the female external genitalia or other injury to the female genital organs whether for cultural or other non-therapeutic reasons." |
| **Type I** | Excision of the prepuce, with or without excision of part or all of the clitoris. Other terms used to describe Type I procedures include circumcision, ritualistic circumcision, sunna, and clitoridectomy. |
| **Type II** | Excision of the clitoris with partial or total excision of the labia minora (Fig. A–1A, B). Other terms used to describe Type II procedures include clitoridectomy, sunna, excision, and circumcision. |

---

*Adapted from Female Genital Mutilation. A Joint WHO/ UNICEF/UNFPA Statement. Geneva, World Health Organization, 1997, p 3.

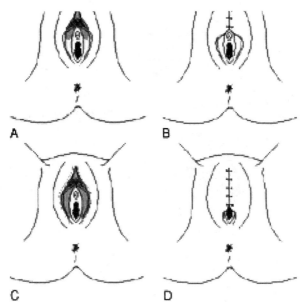

**Figure A–1.** Examples of female genital mutilation. (*A*) Area of tissue removed—Type II FGM; (*B*) Appearance of Type II after suture; (*C*) Area of tissue removed—Type III FGM; (*D*) Appearance of Type III after suture. These figures are examples only; considerable variations occur within FGM types. (Source: Prepared by the Educational Resource Centre of the Women's and Children's Health Care Network, Victoria, Australia, and reproduced with the permission of the Royal Australian and New Zealand College of Obstetricians and Gynaecologists.)

| | |
|---|---|
| **Type III** | Excision of part or all of the external genitalia and stitching/narrowing of the vaginal opening (infibulation) (see Figure A–1*C*, *D*). Other terms used to describe Type III procedures include infibulation, pharaonic circumcision, and Somalian circumcision. |
| **Type IV** | Unclassified: includes any other procedure that falls under the definition of female genital mutilation given above. |

# B

## APPENDIX

# Staging of Gynecologic Cancers

Two professional organizations are devoted to defining the stage of gynecologic cancers. Since 1976, the criteria of the Tumor, Nodes, and Metastases (TNM) Committee of the International Union Against Cancer and the International Federation of Gynecology and Obstetrics (FIGO) have been in agreement for the staging of cancers of the vulva, vagina, cervix, uterus, and ovary. Because the FIGO definitions are more descriptive, they are the ones cited here. In the staging systems shown here, a distinction is made between clinical staging and surgical staging. The diagnosis of cancer cannot be made without a biopsy specimen and histologic examination—in some sense, a surgical procedure. Nonetheless, for those cancers that are clinically staged, information obtained by subsequent surgical treatment does not change the official stage of the cancer. For cancer of the breast, the TNM classification is used, because FIGO does not publish guidelines for this area.

**PEARL: The TNM classification does have some consistency for different cancers. "T" (tumor) is generally designated with numbers 1 to 4 with increasing size. For most gynecologic cancers, N (nodes) is assigned a 0 (zero) for no**

disease in the lymph nodes, 1 for unilateral spread, and 2
for bilateral spread. M stands for distant metastases and is
either absent (0) or present (1).

### VULVAR CARCINOMA—
### SURGICALLY STAGED

  I. Tumor confined to vulva and no larger than 2 cm;
no cancer in lymph nodes
    A. Stromal invasion equal to or less than 1mm
    B. Stromal invasion greater than 1 mm
 II. Tumor confined to vulva but larger than 2 cm; no
cancer in lymph nodes
III. Tumor extension to urethra, vagina, or anus
*and/or* cancer in unilateral groin nodes
IV. Tumor meets stage III requirements plus:
    A. Fixation to bone *and/or* cancer in bilateral
groin nodes
    B. Distant spread (including pelvic nodes)

### VAGINAL CARCINOMA—
### CLINICALLY STAGED

  I. Tumor limited to vaginal wall
 II. Tumor invading adjacent tissue but not to pelvic
side wall
III. Tumor extending to pelvic side wall
IV. A. Tumor extending to rectal or bladder mucosa
or beyond true pelvis
    B. Distant spread

### CERVICAL CARCINOMA—
### CLINICALLY STAGED

  I. A. Tumor not grossly visible—diagnosed only
with magnification
     1. *Depth* less than or equal to 3 mm, *width*
equal to or less than 5 mm
     2. Exceeds IA1 but *depth* less than or equal to
5 mm, *width* equal to or less than 7 mm

    B. Tumor dimension greater than stage IA2 but still confined to cervix

  II. Tumor involving proximal two-thirds of the vagina

    A. No parametrial involvement

    B. Tumor involves parametrial tissues

 III. Tumor extends to lower vagina or pelvic side walls.

    A. No extension to pelvic wall

    B. Extends to pelvic wall and/or all cases with hydronephrosis or non-functioning kidneys unless the condition was pre-existing.

 IV. Tumor has spread beyond pelvis or involves rectum or bladder.

    A. No distant spread beyond adjacent organs

    B. Distant spread

## UTERINE CARCINOMA— SURGICALLY STAGED

For each stage, the grade of tumor must be specified. Grade 1 refers to 5% or less of a nonsquamous solid growth pattern. Grade 2 is 6% to 50% of the same, and Grade 3 is greater than 50%. These grades roughly correspond to well, moderately, and poorly differentiated, respectively.

   I. Tumor confined to the uterus

    A. Tumor confined to *endometrium*

    B. Tumor invasion confined to less than one-half of the *myometrium*

    C. Tumor invasion exceeding one-half of the *myometrium*

  II. Extension to the cervix

    A. Endocervical glands involved only

    B. Cervix involved beyond endocervical glands

 III. Tumor extends beyond uterus and cervix

    A. Tumor invading serosa or adnexa *and/or* positive peritoneal cytology

    B. Tumor spreading to vagina

 IV. Tumor with spread to bowel, bladder or distant sites

    A. Tumor invading bladder or bowel

    B. Distant spread

## FALLOPIAN TUBE
## CARCINOMA—SURGICALLY
## STAGED (ABBREVIATED)

I. Tumor limited to the fallopian tubes
II. Tumor extending to pelvis
III. Peritoneal implants outside the pelvis *and/or* positive retroperitoneal or inguinal nodes
IV. Distant spread

## OVARIAN CARCINOMA—
## SURGICALLY STAGED

I. Growth limited to the ovaries
   A. One ovary
   B. Both ovaries
   C. Tumor on surface of ovary *and/or* ruptured capsule *and/or* malignant ascites or positive peritoneal washings
II. Pelvic extension
   A. Tumor extending to the uterus or tubes
   B. Tumor extending to other pelvic tissues
   C. Tumor as above but also on ovarian capsule and/or malignant ascites or positive peritoneal washings
III. Tumor with peritoneal implants outside the pelvis *and/or* positive retroperitoneal or inguinal nodes
   A. Tumor grossly limited to pelvis with negative nodes but microscopic seeding of peritoneal surface
   B. Peritoneal tumors all equal to or less than 2 cm in diameter with negative nodes
   C. Peritoneal tumor greater than 2 cm *and/or* positive nodes
IV. Distant spread (outside peritoneal cavity)

## BREAST CARCINOMA—
## SURGICALLY STAGED

Tumor size 1 (T1) is 2 cm or less, size 2 is 2 to 5 cm, 3 is greater than 5 cm, and 4 is any extension to chest wall or skin. Node status 0 (N0) is no nodal involvement; 1

## Table B–1. TNM BREAST
## CANCER STAGING

| Stage | Characteristics |
|-------|-----------------|
| Stage I | T1, N0, M0 |
| Stage II | |
| A | T0/T1/T2, N0/N1, M0 |
| B | T3, N0, M0 |
| Stage III | |
| A | T1/T2/T3, N1/N2, M0 |
| B | T1/T2/T3/T4, N0/N1/N2/N3, M0 |
| Stage IV | T1/T2/T3/T4, N0/N1/N2/N3, M1 |

T = tumor, N = node, M = distant metastases.

is involvement of an ipsilateral, movable axillary node; 2 is involvement of an ipsilateral, fixed node; and 3 is involvement of an ipsilateral mammary node. Distant metastases are either absent (M0) or present (M1). Table B-1 lists possible designations for various stages in the TNM classification system.

   I. Tumor 2 cm or less
  II. Tumor >2 cm
     A. Tumor 5 cm or less *and/or* positive ipsilateral axillary nodes
     B. Tumor greater than 5 cm with no positive nodes or distant metastases
 III. Tumor >5cm *or* with fixed axillary nodes
     A. Tumor up to 5 cm with fixed axillary nodes *or* tumor greater than 5 cm with any positive axillary nodes
     B. Metastases to internal mammary nodes *or* extension to chest wall or satellite skin nodule of same breast
 IV. Distant spread

# C

# Dictations of Five Surgeries

Surgical dictations follow a general format:

1. Patient name
2. Date of surgery
3. Date of dictation (hospital bylaws almost always require that the two dates are the same)
4. Preoperative diagnosis
5. Postoperative diagnosis
6. Title of operation
7. Findings
8. Technique (actual description of procedure)
9. Complications
10. Estimated blood loss (some may also mention total input and output)
11. Reference to sponge and needle count (if they are not correct, an intraoperative x-ray study is required to be sure that nothing is inadvertently left behind in the patient)

The following dictations are limited to the "technique" section. "Findings" have been omitted here, because they have to be customized to each patient and are traditionally dictated before "technique." You will notice that occasionally they are referred to in these dictations of technique.

# ABDOMINAL HYSTERECTOMY WITH BILATERAL SALPINGO-OOPHORECTOMY

With the patient under general anesthesia, she was prepped and draped in the usual fashion for an abdominal hysterectomy. A Pfannenstiel abdominal incision was made and then bowel was packed, and a self-retained retractor was placed into the abdomen taking care to avoid the psoas muscles. The pelvis was explored with the findings as above, and the uterus was then grasped over both cornua with a Kocher clamp. The left round ligament was then clamped, divided, and suture ligated with a suture of #0 Vicryl. The vesicouterine peritoneum was then divided in a semicircular fashion over the lower uterine segment. The infundibulopelvic ligament was then skeletonized, and the ureter was identified on the medial leaf of the broad ligament. The infundibulopelvic ligament was then doubly clamped, divided, and suture ligated with a pulley suture of #0 Vicryl and then a free tie of #0 Vicryl. Exactly the same procedure was carried out on the right side.

The bladder was then sharply and bluntly dissected off the lower uterine segment and retracted. The right uterine artery was skeletonized, doubly clamped, divided, and ligated with a Haney suture of #0 Vicryl. Exactly the same thing was done on the left side. The left cardinal ligament was then clamped, followed by the right. Both ligaments were then divided and suture ligated with a Haney suture of #0 Vicryl. The left uterosacral ligament, together with the left lateral apex of the vagina, were then clamped. The same procedure was carried out on the right. The uterus, tubes and ovaries, together with the cervix, were then excised from the patient and handed off the table. Both pedicles were ligated with a Haney suture of #0 Vicryl. The remainder of the cuff was closed with a running, locking suture of #0 Vicryl.

Each of the pedicles was inspected for hemostasis, and small bleeding arterioles were cauterized. The pelvis was then irrigated, and the laparotomy pads and self-retaining retractor were then removed. The fascia was closed with two separate running sutures of #0 Vicryl at either end, meeting in the middle after inspecting the underlying muscle for hemostasis. The subcutaneous tissue was dry, and the skin was closed using staples. There were no intraoperative complications. Estimated blood loss was 400 mL. Sponge and needle counts were correct at the end of case. The patient was awakened and returned to the recovery room, alert and in good condition.

## VAGINAL HYSTERECTOMY

With the patient under general anesthesia, she was prepped and draped in the usual fashion in the dorsal lithotomy position for a vaginal hysterectomy. A pelvic exam under anesthesia was performed, and then the cervix was exposed and grasped on the anterior and posterior lips with single-tooth tenacula. A circumferential incision around the cervix was made with a knife. The anterior and posterior cul-de-sacs were then entered with a combination of blunt and sharp dissection. The left uterosacral ligament was then clamped, divided, and suture ligated with a Haney suture of #0 Vicryl. Exactly the same was done on the patient's right. The right cardinal ligament was then clamped, divided, and suture ligated with a Haney suture of #0 Vicryl. The same was done with the left cardinal ligament. The left uterine artery was then clamped, divided, and suture ligated with a Haney suture of #0 Vicryl as was the right. At this point, the fundus of the uterus was delivered posteriorly through the introitus. The uterine cornua, incorporating the ovarian suspensory ligament, round ligament, and fallopian tube, were then clamped on either side, and the uterus was then excised from the patient. Each of these pedicles was ligated with a pulley suture of #0 Vicryl and then a free tie of #0 Vicryl.

The ovaries were visualized and found to be normal. Each of the pedicles was inspected for hemostasis, which was good. The visceral peritoneum was reapproximated using a purse-string suture of 2–0 Vicryl. The vaginal cuff was closed by placing a figure of 8 suture of #0 Vicryl in either corner and then closing the remainder with a running, locking suture of #0

Vicryl. Hemostasis was good. Estimated blood loss was 200 mL. There were no intraoperative complications. Sponge and needle counts were correct at the end of the case. The patient was awakened and returned to the recovery room, alert and in good condition.

## DIAGNOSTIC LAPAROSCOPY

With the patient under general anesthesia, she was prepped and draped in the dorsal lithotomy position in the usual fashion for a diagnostic laparoscopy. The bladder was straight catheterized, and a pelvic exam with the findings as above was performed. A sponge stick was placed into the vagina to permit uterine manipulation. A small incision was then made in the umbilicus, through which a Veress needle was placed. No gas was aspirated, and water flowed freely through the needle. Carbon dioxide gas for a total of 3 liters was then placed under high pressure through the needle. The incision was then enlarged, the needle removed, and an 11-mm laparoscopy sheath with trocar in place was then inserted into the abdomen. The trocar was removed, and the laparoscope was then inserted. It was indeed within the peritoneal cavity. At this point, a second incision was made, transversely, in the midline at the level of the pubic hair line, through which a 5-mm laparoscopy sleeve with trocar in place was inserted into the peritoneal cavity while watching the tip through the laparoscope.

The trocar was removed, and a steel probe was inserted. The pelvis and abdomen were then explored with the findings as above. At this point, the probe was removed and then the laparoscope. The carbon dioxide gas was allowed to escape through both sleeves, and they were then removed. The umbilical incision was closed with a figure-of-8 suture of #0 Vicryl in the fascia and two simple interrupted sutures of 2–0 plain in the skin. The lower incision was closed with a simple suture of 2–0 plain. The wounds were cleaned and dressed with adhesive bandages. The sponge stick was removed from the vagina, and the patient was awakened and returned to the recovery room alert and in good condition. The estimated blood loss was perhaps 10 mL. There were no intraoperative complications. Sponge and needle counts were correct at the end of the case.

## DILATION AND CURETTAGE
## WITH HYSTEROSCOPY

Under intravenous sedation, the patient was prepped and draped in the dorsal lithotomy position in the usual fashion for a dilation and curettage (D&C). A pelvic exam was performed, and then the cervix was exposed and grasped on the anterior lip with a single-tooth tenaculum. A paracervical block, using 4 mL of 1% lidocaine, was placed at 3:00 and 9:00 after aspiration to be sure that the needle was not in a vessel. At this point, an endocervical curettage was performed using a kevorkian curette. The uterus was then sounded to 8 cm and dilated to 9 mm. A hysteroscope using glycine as a distending medium was then inserted with the findings as above. A polyp forceps was then introduced, which obtained minimal tissue. The uterus was then sharply curetted over all surfaces. At this point, all of the instruments in the uterus were removed, and the tenaculum was taken off the cervix. The cervix was inspected for hemostasis, which was good. The speculum was removed and the patient was awakened and returned directly to the floor, alert and in good condition. The estimated blood loss was perhaps 10 mL. There were no intraoperative complications. The sponge count was correct at the end of the case.

## BURCH PROCEDURE
## WITH INSERTION OF
## SUPRAPUBIC CATHETER

With the patient under general anesthesia, she was prepped and draped in dorsal lithotomy position in the usual fashion for a Burch procedure. A Pfannenstiel abdominal incision was made 3 cm above the symphysis. The space of Retzius was entered, and the vesicovaginal fascia and Cooper's ligament were bluntly and sharply dissected free of adipose tissue. The surgeon placed his left hand inside the vagina to facilitate suture placement and identify the bladder neck. 100 mL of indigo carmine dye was placed into the bladder, and the Foley was then clamped to help demonstrate the bladder edges. A double throw of 2–0 Gore-Tex suture was then placed into the vesicovaginal fascia 1 cm to the right of the urethra at the level of the bladder neck. A second double-throw suture of 2–0 Gore-Tex was placed 1 cm to the right of the urethra, 1 cm distal to the first suture. Exactly the same procedure was repeated on left side. At this point, the left distal suture was placed into the medial aspect of the left Cooper's ligament.

The proximal left suture was placed into Cooper's ligament 1 cm lateral to the first suture. The same procedure was followed on the right side. The sutures were then tied down by the assistant in sequence while the surgeon helped to support the bladder neck with his vaginal hand, starting with the right proximal, then right distal, left distal, and left proximal. Good support of the bladder neck and proximal urethra was obtained, although the surgeon could still insert his fifth digit between the urethra and the back of the symphysis.

An additional 300 mL of indigo carmine dye was placed into the bladder. A stab incision was made in the midline 3 cm above the Pfannenstiel incision. A Microvasive suprapubic catheter with trocar in place was then inserted through the stab incision in the skin and then through the fascia and into the bladder while watching the tip. The trocar was removed, and the catheter was then locked into position and sewn to the skin by a 3–0 silk. The bladder was then allowed to drain through both catheters. The fascia was closed with two separate running sutures of #0-Dexon starting at either end and meeting in the middle. The subcutaneous tissue was dry, and the skin was closed using staples. The wound was cleaned and dressed, and the catheter was taped into position. The patient was then awakened and returned to the recovery room alert and in good condition. Estimated blood loss was 75 mL. There were no intraoperative complications. Sponge and needle counts were correct at the end of the case.

# Index

*Page numbers with *f* indicate figures; those with *t* indicate tables.

Abdominal hysterectomy, 190–194, *192*
  with bilateral salpingo-oophorectomy, 221–222
Abortion, 59–64, 67. *See also* Miscarriage
  cost of, 67
  medical methods of, 63
  safety of, 64
Abscess, Bartholin duct, 74–76
Abused women, complaints of, 7
Acquired immunodeficiency syndrome (AIDS), 113, 115
Adenocarcinoma, 126
Adenomatous hyperplasia, 168
Adenomyosis, 163–164
Adnexa, 8
AIDS (acquired immunodeficiency syndrome), 113, 115
Alendronate (Fosamax) for osteoporosis, 149
Amenorrhea, 64
Anatomy, gynecologic, 3–6, 4f, 5f, 6f
Androgen replacement, 142
Anorexia nervosa, 16
Anovulation, 21, 25, 152
  adenomyosis, 163–164
  clomiphene citrate, 158–159
  endometriosis, 161
    diagnosis, 161–162
  female genital tract abnormalities, 159–161
  gonadotropin treatment, 159
  hypothalamic, 22
  treatment, 162–163
Anterior colporrhaphy, 96
Anus, 4, 4f, 5f
Arteries, 6f
Asherman's syndrome, 64
Atrophic vaginitis, 70
AutoPap 200, 131
Azithymidine (AZT) for human immunodeficiency virus (HIV), 117

Bacterial vaginosis, 72, 101t

Bartholin duct abscess, 74–75
  excision of gland, 76
  incision and drainage, 75
  marsupialization, 75
Bartholin's gland, 5*f*, 6*f*
Basal body temperature in assessing ovulation, 153
Basal cell, 165
Benign uterine abnormalities, 25
Bethesda system, 132, 133*t*
Bilateral salpingo-oophorectomy, 190–194
  abdominal hysterectomy with, 221–222
Bimanual (two-handed) exam, 8
Biopsy
  breast, 178
  cone, 139–140
  endometrial, 26, 141, 153–154
  thin-needle aspiration, 177
Birth control pill. *See* Combination oral contraceptive pill
Bladder, overactive, 91
Bladder prolapse, 87, 88
Bladder training, 96
Bleeding
  excessive, 24–27, 25*f*
  first-trimester, 27–29, 28*t*
  postmenopausal, 149–150
Body of uterus, 6*f*
Bone mineral density (BMD), 148
BRCA1, 178
BRCA2, 178
Breast aspiration, 177
Breast biopsy, 178
Breast cancer, 39, 218–219, 219*t*
  diagnosis of
    aspiration, 177
    biopsy, 178
    genetics and prevention, 178–179
    mammography, 176–177
    self-examination, 178
    thin-needle aspiration biopsy, 177
  treatment of, 179–180
Breast development, 16
  Marshall and Tanner's classification of, 17, 17*t*
Breast disease, history and physical examination, 174–176,
    *175*
Breast examination, 7
Breastfeeding, 40
Breast self-examination, 178
Brenner tumors, 171
Broad ligament, 6*f*

Bromocriptine (Parlodel) for galactorrhea, 81
Burch procedure, 96, 200–202
  with insertion of suprapubic catheter, 224–225

CA-125, 172
Cabergoline (Dostinex) for galactorrhea, 81
Cancer
  breast, 218–219, 219*t*
  cervical, 125, 167, 216–217
  endometrial, 21, 25, 26, 141
  fallopian tube, 218
  ovarian, 218
  risk of, 39
  squamous cell, 126
  staging of, 215–219
  uterine, 217
  vaginal, 216
  vulvar, 166, 216
*Candida* vulvovaginitis, 68–70
  treatment of, 69*t*
Carbohydrate intolerance, 40
Carbon dioxide laser, 187
Carcinoma. *See* Cancer
Cardinal ligament, 193
Cardiovascular disease, risk of, 39
Cerebrovascular accidents, risk of, 39
Cervical cap, 55
Cervical carcinoma, 125, 167, 216–217
  squamous, *129*
Cervical condylomata, 128–129
Cervical cytology, 130–131
  Bethesda system, 132, 133*t*
  pap smear technique, 131–132
Cervical incompetence, 140
Cervical intraepithelial neoplasia, biology of, *129,* 129–
      130
Cervical portio, 8
Cervix, 4, 5, 5*f*
  inspection of, in pelvic examination, 7–8
  microscopic anatomy of, 125–126
  of uterus, 6*f*
Chancroid, 101*t*
Chemotherapy, 180
Chlamydia, 48, 102*t*
Choriocarcinoma, 173
Circumcision, female, 10–11
Clitoris, 3, 4, 4*f,* 5*f*
Colporraphy, anterior, 96
Colposcopy, 125–140, 134–135

Combination oral-contraceptive pill, 30–41
  advantages, 40
  choosing, 31–32, 33–35*t*
  cost, 41
  directions for use, 36–38
  disadvantages, 40
  effectiveness, 66*t*
  hormonal structure of, 31, 31*f*, 32*f*
  "morning-after," 41
  progestin implants (Norplant), 42–44
  progestin injections (Depo-Provera), 42
  progestin-only, 41–42
  safety, 38–40, 65*t*
Committee of the International Union Against Cancer, 215
Complete blood count (CBC), 203
Complete miscarriage, 27
Condoms, 50–51
  female, 51
Condyloma acuminatum, 102*t*
Condylomata, 165
  cervical, 128–129
  external, 128, 165
  treatment of, 128–129
  vaginal, 128
Cone biopsy, 139–140
Continuous estrogen and cyclic progestin, 145
Continuous incontinence, 91
Contraception, 30
  abortion, 59–64, 67
  cervical cap, 55
  combination oral pill, 30–41
  condoms, 50–51
  diaphragm, 51–55, 53*f*, 54*f*
  dilation and evacuation, 60–63
  effectiveness, 66*t*, 67
  female sterilization, 55–58
  intrauterine device, 44–49
  male sterilization, 59
  periodic abstinence, 55
  safety, 65*t*, 67
  spermicides, 49–50
Cooper's ligament, 201
Corpus luteum, 6*f*, 14
Cryosurgery, 136
Cushing's syndrome, 84
Cyclic estrogen and progestin, 145
Cystadenomas, mucinous, 171
Cystic hyperplasia, 168
Cystocele, 87

Cystometry, 94–95
Cystoscopy, 167

D&C (dilation and curettage), 26, 199–200
  with hysteroscopy, 224
D&E (dilation and evacuation), 60–63
Dehydroepiandrosterone sulfate (DHEAS) and hirsutism,
  82–83
Depo-Provera, 20, 42
Depression and decreased libido, 79
Detrusor instability, 90–91, 95, 96
DHEAS (dehydroepiandrosterone sulfate) and hirsutism,
  82–83
Diabetes and vulvar neuropathy, 70
Diagnostic laparoscopy, 223–224
Diaphragm, 18, 51–55, 53f, 54f
Dilation and curettage (D&C), 26, 199–200
  with hysteroscopy, 224
Dilation and evacuation (D&E), 60–63
Douches, 19–20
Dysgerminoma, 171–172
Dysmenorrhea, 20–21
  treatment of, 20–21

Ectopic pregnancy, 28–29, 47, 60
Electrical stimulation, 99
Electrosurgical devices, 188
Embolism, pulmonary, 208–209
Embryo transfer, 160
Endocrinology. *See* Reproductive endocrinology
Endocrinopathies, 156
Endodermal sinus tumor, 172
Endometrial biopsy, 26, 141
  in assessing ovulation, 153–154
Endometrial carcinoma, 21, 25, 26, 141
Endometrial hyperplasia, 25
Endometrial neoplasms, 168–169
Endometrial polyps, 26
Endometriosis, 20, 161
  as cause of dyspareunia, 74
  diagnosis of, 161–162
Endometrium, 6f
  atrophies of, 149
Enterocele, 87, 89
Epidural narcotics, 206–207
Epithelial cell tumors, 171
Estrogen, 13, 14
Evista (raloxifene), 142–143, 145
Excessive bleeding, 24–27, 25f

External condylomata, 128

Fallopian tubes, 5, 5*f*, 6*f*
    carcinoma of, 218
Female circumcision, 10–11
Female genital mutilation, 10–11
    classification of, by World Health Organization (WHO),
        213–214, *214*
Female genital tract abnormalities for anovulation, 159–161
Female sterilization, 55–58
Feminine hygiene
    douches, 19–20
    sanitary napkins and tampons, 18–19
Fertilization, 13, 160
    of ovum, 6*f*
FIGO (International Federation of Gynecology and Obstet-
        rics), 215
Fimbriae, 5, 6*f*
First-trimester bleeding, 27–29
    evaluation of, 28*t*
Fistulas, urinary tract, 91
Fitz-Hugh-Curtis syndrome, 117
Fluorescent treponemal antibody test (FTA-ABS), 121–122
Follicle-stimulating hormone (FSH), 14, 30
Follicular phase, 13
FSH (follicle-stimulating hormone), 14, 30
Fundus of uterus, 6*f*
Fungal infections, 68–70, 69*t*

Galactorrhea, 79–82, *80*
Gallbladder disease, 40
Gamete intrafallopian tube transfer (GIFT), 161
Genital herpes infection, 111, *112*
    diagnosis, 113
    symptoms, 112–113
    treatment, 113, 114*t*
Germ cell tumors, 171–172
Gestational trophoblastic disease, 173
    hydatidiform mole, 173–174
    invasive mole and choriocarcinoma, 174
GiFT (gamete intrafallopian tube transfer), 161
Gonadoblastoma, 172
Gonadotropin-releasing hormone (GnRH), 14
Gonadotropin treatment for anovulation, 159
Gonorrhea, 48, 103*t*
GnRH (gonadotropin-releasing hormone), 14
Granuloma, 103*t*

hCG (human chorionic gonadotropin) levels, 281

Heart disease, 22
Hepatitis B, 103*t*, 108, *109*
  symptoms, 108–110
  vaccine for, 111
Hepatitis e antigen (HBeAG), 108
Hepatitis surface antigen (HBsAG), 108
Herpes simplex, 104*t*
Herpes simplex virus (HSV)-1, 111
Herpes simplex virus (HSV)-2, 111
High-grade squamous intraepithelial lesion (HGSIL), 136
Hirsutism, 82–84, *83*, 156
History, 6–7, 174–176, *175*
HIV. See Human immunodeficiency virus (HIV) infection
Home ovulation detection kits, 15
Horizontal incision, 190–191
Hormone replacement therapy (HRT), 22, 142–143
  common regimens, 145
  disease-preventive effects of, 143, 144*t*, 145
  specific preparations, 145, 146*t*, 147
Hot flashes, 141
HPV. See Human papillomavirus (HPV)
HRT. *See* Hormone replacement therapy
HSV (herpes simplex virus)-1, 111
HSV (herpes simplex virus)-2, 111
Human chorionic gonadotropin (hCG) levels, 28
Human immunodeficiency virus (HIV) infection, 100, 104*t*,
      108, 113, 115
  diagnosis, 115–116
  symptoms, 115
  treatment, 116–117
Human papillomavirus (HPV), 125
  transmission and management, 126–127
HUMI uterine manipulator, 197
Hydatidiform mole, 173–174
Hymen, 4, 4*f*
Hypercholesterolemia, 39
Hyperprolactinemia, 80
Hypothalamic anovulation, 22
Hypothalamus, 14
Hysterectomy, 140
  abdominal, 190–194, *192*
  vaginal, 89, 194–196, *195*, 222–223
Hysterosalpingogram, 154–155
Hysteroscopy, 26–27, 156, 199–200
  dilation and curettage (D&C) with, 224
Hysterosonogram, 26

Ibuprofen, 20, 21
Immature cystic teratoma, 172

Incontinence
  continuous, 91
  overflow, 91
Infertility. *See also* Male infertility
  evaluation of, 152
    assessment of female genital tract, 154–156
    assessment of ovulation, 152–154
    endocrinopathies, 156
    semen quality, 152, 153*t*
  treatment of, 156–161
Infibulation, 213
Intercourse, pain on, 74
International Federation of Gynecology and Obstetrics
        (FIGO), 215
Intrauterine device, 44–49
  cost, 49
  disadvantages, 48–49
  effectiveness, 66*t*
  insertion and removal, 45–46, 46*f*
  safety, 47–48, 65*t*
Introitus, 3–4
Invasive mole and choriocarcinoma, 174
*In vitro* fertilization IVF) for anovulation, 159–161
IUD. *See* Intrauterine device
IVF (*in vitro* fertilization) for anovulation, 159–161

Jock itch, 68

Kaposi's sarcoma, 115
Kegel exercises, 96–97

Labia majora, 3
Labia minora, 4
Labium majus, 4*f*, 5*f*
Labium minus, 4*f*, 5*f*
Laminaria, 60–61
Laparoscopy, 56–57, 156, 196–199, *197*
  diagnostic, 223–224
  instruments for, 185, 187
Large loop excision of the transformation zone (LLETZ), 137
Lasers, 138–139
  and electrosurgical devices, 187–188
LeFort operation, 89
Levlen, 32
Levonorgestrel implants (Norplant), 20
LGSIL (low-grade squamous intraepithelial lesion), 136
LH. *See* Luteinizing hormone (LH)
Libido, decreased, 79
Lice *(Phthirus pubis)*, 105*t*

Lichen sclerosis, 70, 165
Lichen simplex chronicus, 70
Linear salpingostomy, 29
LLETZ (large loop excision of the transformation zone, 137
Loop electrosurgical excision procedure, 136–138
Low-grade squamous intraepithelial lesion (LGSIL), 136
Low-pressure urethra, 91
Lumpectomy, 179–180
Luteal phase, 14
Luteinizing hormone (LH), 14, 30
    surge of, 14, 15
Lymphogranuloma inguinale, 105*t*

Male infertility, 157. *See also* Infertility
    donor sperm, 157–158
    efforts to improve sperm delivery, 157
    improving semen quality, 157
Male sterilization, 59
Malignancy, 25
Mammography, 176–177
Marshall-Marchetti-Krantz procedure, 96, 200
Marsupialization, 75
Mastectomy, 180
Maylard incision, 190, 191
Medroxyprogesterone (Depo-Provera), 20
Melanoma, 165
Menarche, 12, 15, 16
Menopause, 141–150
    hormone replacement therapy for, 142–143
        common regimens, 145
        disease-preventive effects of, 143, 144*t*, 145
        specific preparations, 145, 146*t*, 147
    osteoporosis in, 147–149
    postmenopausal bleeding in, 149–150
    premature ovarian failure in, 150
Menorrhagia, 168
Menses, 12
Menstrual cycle, 12–15, 15*f*
    purpose of, 12
Menstruation
    infrequent, 21–22, 22*f*, 23*t*
    painful, 20–21
Methotrexate, 29
Midcycle spotting, 168
Minilaparotomy, 56–57
Miscarriage, 27–28, 48. *See also* Abortion
    terminology, 27
Mittelschmerz, 13
Molluscum, 105*t*

Mons pubis, 3, 4*f*
Morning-after pill, 41
Mucinous cystadenomas, 171
*Mycoplasma hominis,* 117
Myocardial infarction, risk of, 39
Myomectomy, 170
Myometrial neoplasms, 169–170
Myometrium, 6*f*

Naproxen sodium, 20
Neoplasms
    endometrial, 168–169
    myometrial, 169–170
Neurosyphilis, 124
Nonylphenoxypolyethoxyethanol (nonoxynol 9), 49
Nordette, 32
Norinyl 1/35, 32, 33*t*, 36
Norplant, 20, 42–44, 43*f*, 66*t*

Obstructive devices, 99
Oocytes, 13
    maturation, 160
    retrieval, 160
Oral contraceptives, 20, 30–41, 33–35*t*
    effectiveness, 66*t*
    safety, 65*t*
Ortho-Cept, 32, 35*t*
Ortho Cyclen, 35*t*, 36
Ortho-Novum, 31, 32, 33*t*, 36
Ortho Tri-Cyclen, 35*t*, 36
Os, 4, 8
Osteopenia, 148
Osteoporosis, 22, 143, 147–149
Ovarian carcinoma, 218
Ovarian ligament, 6*f*
Ovarian neoplasms, 171
    diagnosis, 172–173
    epithelial cell tumors, 171
    germ cell tumors, 171–172
    stromal cell tumors, 171
Ovaries, 5, 5*f*, 6*f*
Overactive bladder, 91
Overflow incontinence, 91
Oviducts, 5
Ovulation, 13, 14
    assessment of, in evaluation of infertility, 152–154

Paget's disease, 166

Pain
  on intercourse, 74
  in menstruation, 20–21
  pelvic, 84
  postoperative relief, 206–207
Papanicolaou, George, 130
Papanicolaou smears, 8, 125, 130–131
  follow-up of abnormal, 132–135
  technique, 131–132
PapNet, 131
Parlodel for galactorrhea, 81
Patient-controlled analgesia (PCA), 206, 207
PCA (patient-controlled analgesia), 206, 207
PCOS (polycystic ovarian syndrome), 23–24
Pelvic examination
  bimanual (two-handed), 8
  inspection of vulva, vagina, and cervix, 7–8
  recording, 9
  rectal-vaginal, 8
  steps in making more bearable, 9–10
Pelvic inflammatory disease (PID), 47, 106*f*, 106*t*, 117
  complications, 119
  diagnosis, 118
  symptoms, 117–118
  treatment, 118–119, 119*t*
Pelvic masses as cause of dyspareunia, 74
Pelvic muscle exercises, 96–97
Pelvic pain, 84
Perihepatitis, 117
Perineum, 3
Periodic abstinence, 55
Pfannenstiel's abdominal incision, 190, 191, 221, 224, 225
Physical examination, 174–176, *175*
PID. *See* Pelvic inflammatory disease (PID)
Pill. *See also* Combination oral-contraceptive pill
  morning-after, 41
  progestin-only, 41–42
*Pneumocystis carinii* pneumonia, 115
Pneumonia, *Pneumocystis carinii*, 115
Polycystic ovarian syndrome (PCOS), 23–24
Polyglycolic acid sutures, 208
Polyps, 25
Portio vaginalis cervicis, 8
Postcoital test, 155–156
Posterior colporrhaphy, 88
Posterior fourchette, 4
Postmenopausal bleeding, 149–150
Postoperative complications, 208–209
Postoperative orders, 205–206

Postoperative pain relief, 206–207
Post-void residual, 93
Potassium-titanyl-phosphate (KTP) laser, 188
Pregnancy, 21
  ectopic, 28–29, 47, 60
Premature ovarian failure, 150
Premenstrual syndrome, 77–78
Preoperative considerations, 203–204
Procidentia, 87, 89
Progesterone, 13
  level, 28
    in assessing ovulation, 153
Progestin
  supplementation, 142
  withdrawal, 22
Progestin implants. *See* Norplant
Progestin injections. *See* Depo-Provera
Progestin-only pill, 41–42
Prolactin, 21
  levels, 81
Prolapse
  bladder, 87, 88
  definitions, 87, 88*t*
  rectal, 88
  surgical treatment
    enterocele, 89
    rectocele, 88
    uterine, 89
  symptoms, 88
  uterine, 87, 89
Prostaglandin E in abortion, 63
Protease inhibitors, 116–117
Puberty, 15–18, 16*t*
  abnormalities in, 17–18
Pubic hair, 3
  Marshall and Tanner's classification of growth of, 17, 17*t*
Pubic lice, 100, 108
Pulmonary angiography, 209
Pulmonary embolism, 208–209

Q-tip test, 93

Radiation treatment, 179–180
Raloxifene (Evista), 142–143, 145
Rapid plasma reagin (RPR), 121
Rectal herniation, 87
Rectal prolapse, 88
Rectal-vaginal exam, 8
Rectocele, 88

Rectum, 5f
Reproductive endocrinology, 151–164
  evaluation of infertile couple, 152
    assessment of female genital tract, 154–156
    assessment of ovulation, 152–154
    endocrinopathies, 156
    semen quality, 152, 153t
Retropubic urethral suspensions, 96, 200
Reverse transcriptase inhibitors (RTI), 116–117
Rh immune globulin (RhoGAM), 28
Rh-negative women, 28
RhoGam (rh immune globulin), 28
Ritonavir (Norvir) for human immunodeficiency virus (HIV),
    117
Round ligament, 6f
RPR (rapid plasma reagin), 121
Rubin cannula, 197
Rugae, 6f

Salpingectomy, partial, 29
Salpingostomy, linear, 29
Sanitary napkins and tampons, 18–19
Saquinavir (Invirase) for human immunodeficiency virus
    (HIV), 117
Sarcomas, 170
Scabies *(Sarcoptes scabiei)*, 100, 106t, 108
Scarpa's fascia, 190
Selective estrogen receptor modulators (SERMs), 142
Semen. *See also* Sperm
  charactistics of normal, 152, 153t
  quality of
    in evaluation of infertility, 152, 153t
    improving quality of, 157
Serial ultrasonography in assessing ovulation, 154
SERMs (selective estrogen receptor modulators), 142
Sertoli-Leydig cell tumors, 171
Sexually transmitted diseases (STDs), 18, 51, 100, 101–107t, 108
  diagnosis, 110, 111t
  genital herpes infection, 111, *112*
    diagnosis, 113
    symptoms, 112–113
    treatment, 113, 114t
  hepatitis B, 108, *109*
    symptoms, 108–110
  human immunodeficiency virus (HIV) infection, 113, 115
    diagnosis, 115–116
    symptoms, 115
    treatment, 116–117
  pelvic inflammatory disease (PID), 117

Sexually transmitted diseases (STDs)—*Continued*
    complications, 119
    diagnosis, 118
    symptoms, 117–118
    treatment, 118–119, 119*t*
    prevention, 110–111
Smead-Jones suture technique, 208
Smoking, 39
Space of Retzius, 224
Speculum, 7–8, 9
Sperm, 6. *See* also Semen
    donor, 157–158
    efforts to improve delivery of, 157
Spermicides, 49–50
Squamous cell carcinoma, 126, 165
Squamous intraepithelial lesions, treatment of, 136–140
    cone biopsy, 139–140
    cryosurgery, 136
    hysterectomy, 140
    laser, 138–139
    loop electrosurgical excision procedure, 136–138
*Staphylococcus aureus* in toxic shock syndrome, 76
STDs. *See* Sexually transmitted diseases (STDs)
Sterilization
    female, 55–58
    male, 59
Steroid rebound dermatitis, 72
Strawberry cervix, 73
Stress incontinence, 90, 95–96
Stromal cell tumors, 171
Submucous myomas, 25, 26
Sunday Start method, 36
Suprapubic catheter, Burch procedure with insertion of,
    224–225
Surgical consent, 204–205
Surgical dictations, 220–225
Surgical instruments, materials, and techniques, 183, 184*t*,
    185–189
Surgical technique, 189
Syphilis, 107*t*, 120
    cardiovascular, 124
    complications, 123–124
    congenital, 124
    diagnosis, 121–122
    latent, 123
    mucocutaneous, 123–124
    osseous (bone), 124
    symptoms, 120–121
    tertiary, 123–124

treatment, 122, 122*t*
visceral, 124

Tampon, retained, 76
Testosterone and hirsutism, 82–83
Thin-needle aspiration biopsy, 177
Thromboembolic disease (TED) hose, 203–204
Thyroid-stimulating hormone (TSH), 21
Tinea, 68
Tinea cruris, 69
TNM (Tumor, Nodes, and Metastases, 215–216
Toxic shock syndrome, 19, 76
Transitional cell tumors, 171
Transvaginal ultrasound, 26
*Treponema pallidum*, 120
Trichomonas, 73
Trichomoniasis, 72, 107*t*
Tri-Levlen, 32, 34*t*
Triphasil, 32, 35*t*
TSH (thyroid-stimulating hormone) , 21
Tubal ligations, 56–58, 65*t*, 66*t*
Tubal obstruction, 152, 159
Tumor, Nodes, and Metastases (TNM), 215–216

Ultrasound, in assessment of ovulation, 154
   in ectopic pregnancy, 28
   in PCOS, 23
Urethra, 4
   low-pressure, 91
Urethral meatus, 3, 5*f*
Urethral opening, 4*f*
Urethral patch, 99
Urethral pressure measurements, 95
Urethrocele, 87
Urethrocystocopy, 95
Urge incontinence, 90–91, 95, 96
Urinalysis, 93
Urinary bladder, 5*f*
Urinary incontinence, 89–90
   diagnostic workup, 91
      advanced testing, 93–95
      history and voiding log, 92
      physical examination, 92
      simple tests, 93
   treatment, 95–96, 97–98*t*, 99
   types, 90–91
Urinary luteinizing hormone (LH) surge in assessing ovulation, 153
Urine pregnancy test, 203

Uroflowmetry, 95
Uterine carcinoma, 217
Uterine neoplasms, 167
    endometrial, 168–169
    myometrial, 169–170
    sarcomas, 170
Uterine prolapse, 87, 89
Uterosacral ligament, 193–194
Uterus, 5*f*

Vaccine, hepatitis B, 111
Vagina, 4, 5*f*, 6*f*
    inspection of, in pelvic examination, 7–8
Vaginal carcinoma, 216
Vaginal condylomata, 128
Vaginal discharge, 72–74, 73*t*
    Bartholin duct abscess, 74–75
        excision of gland, 76
        incision and drainage, 75
        marsupialization, 75
    pain on intercourse (dyspareunia), 74
    retained tampon, 76
    toxic shock syndrome, 76
Vaginal electrical resistance in assessing ovulation, 154
Vaginal hemorrhage, 26–27
Vaginal hysterectomy, 89, 194–196, *195*, 222–223
Vaginal introitus, 89
Vaginal opening, 4*f*
Vaginal spotting, 14
Vaginal suppositories, 49–50
Vaginitis, atrophic, 70
Vasectomy, 59
Veins, 6*f*
Venous thromboembolism, risk of, 39
Venous thrombosis prophylaxis, 203
Veress needle, 198
Vertical midline incision, 190
Vestibulitis, 70
VIN (vulvar intraepithelial neoplasia), 70, 128, 165–166
Voiding log, 92
Vulva, 3, 19
    inspection of, in pelvic examination, 7–8
Vulvar cancer, 166, 216
Vulvar intraepithelial neoplasia (VIN), 70, 128, 165–166
Vulvar irritation
    causes of, 70–72
    fungal infections, 68–70, 69*t*
Vulvar lesions, 128, 165–166
Vulvar neoplasms, 165–166

Vulvar neuropathy and diabetes, 70
Vulvar psoriasis, 70
Vulvocandidiasis, 70
Vulvodynia, 70

World Health Organization (WHO), classification of female
    genital mutilation, 213–214, *214*
Wound dehiscence, 208

Yeast infections, 72
Yolk sac tumor, 172
Yttrium-aluminum-garnet (YAG) laser, 188

Zidovudine (ZDV) for human immunodeficiency virus (HIV),
    117
ZIFT (zygote intrafallopian tube transfer), 161
Zygote intrafallopian tube transfer (ZIFT), 161

## DATE DUE

| | | | |
|---|---|---|---|
| | | | |
| | | | |
| | | | |
| | | | |
| | | | |
| | | | |
| | | | |
| | | | |
| | | | |
| | | | |
| | | | |
| | | | |
| | | | |
| | | | |
| | | | |

Demco, Inc. 38-293